Professionalism in Mental Healthcare

Experts, Expertise and Expectations

D1231101

Professionalism in Mental Healthcare

Experts, Expertise and Expectations

Edited by

Dinesh Bhugra
Institute of Psychiatry, King's College London

Amit Malik
Hampshire Partnership NHS Foundation Trust

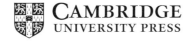

CAMBRIDGE
UNIVERSITY PRESS

CAMBRIDGE UNIVERSITY PRESS
Cambridge, New York, Melbourne, Madrid, Cape Town, Singapore,
São Paulo, Delhi, Dubai, Tokyo, Mexico City

Cambridge University Press
The Edinburgh Building, Cambridge CB2 8RU, UK

Published in the United States of America by Cambridge University
Press, New York

www.cambridge.org
Information on this title: www.cambridge.org/9780521131766

First published 2011

Printed in the United Kingdom at the University Press, Cambridge

*A catalogue record for this publication is available from the
British Library*

Library of Congress Cataloguing in Publication data
Professionalism in mental healthcare : experts, expertise and
expectations / edited by Dinesh Bhugra, Amit Malik.
   p. ; cm.
Includes bibliographical references and index.
ISBN 978-0-521-13176-6 (pbk.)
1. Psychiatry – Practice.   2. Mental health services.   I. Bhugra,
Dinesh.   II. Malik, Amit.
[DNLM: 1. Psychiatry.   2. Professional Competence.   3.
Professional Role.   4. Quality Assurance, Health Care. WM 100]
RC440.8.P76   2010
616.89023 – dc22   2010030220

ISBN 978-0-521-13176-6 Paperback

Contents

Contributors

Robert Adler
Psychiatrist and President of the Medical
Board of Victoria
Melbourne, Australia

Dinesh Bhugra
Professor of Mental Health and Cultural
Diversity
Institute of Psychiatry, King's College
London
London, UK

Sharon Brownie
Royal Australian and New Zealand College
of Psychiatrists
Melbourne
Victoria, Australia

Kenneth Busch
Psychiatrist
Chicago, IL
USA

Julian Freidin
Royal Australian and New Zealand College
of Psychiatrists
Melbourne
Victoria, Australia

Susham Gupta
Consultant Psychiatrist
East London Foundation NHS Trust
Assertive Outreach Team – City &
Hackney
London, UK

Helen Herrman
Professor of Psychiatry, Orygen Youth
Health Research Centre
Centre for Youth Mental Health
The University of Melbourne
Victoria, Australia

James W. Holsinger, Jr
Professor, Department of Health Services
Management
College of Public Health
University of Kentucky
Lexington, KY
USA

Gillian Lewando Hundt
Professor, School of Health and Social
Studies
University of Warwick
Coventry, UK

Sir Donald Irvine
Former President of the General Medical
Council
Morpeth
Northumberland, UK

Vikram Jha
Senior Lecturer
Medical Education Unit
University of Leeds
Leeds, UK

Neil Johnson
Associate Clinical Professor
Institute of Clinical Education
Medical School Building
University of Warwick
Coventry, UK

Amit Malik
Associate Medical Director and Consultant
Psychiatrist
Hampshire Partnership NHS Foundation
Trust
Hampshire, UK

H. Steven Moffic
Professor, Department of Psychiatry and
Behavioral Medicine and Department of

Family and Community Medicine
Medical College of Wisconsin
Milwaukee, WI
USA

Jonathan Montgomery
Professor, School of Law
University of Southampton
Highfield
Southampton, UK

Katinka Morton
Director of Postgraduate Training for
North Western Mental Health
The Royal Melbourne Hospital
Melbourne, Australia

Robert A. Murden
Director, Geriatric Medicine
Professor of Clinical Internal Medicine
OSU Internal Medicine at Morehouse
Columbus, OH
USA

David W. Page
Professor of Surgery
Department of Surgery
Baystate Medical Center
Springfield, MA
USA

Vikram Patel
Professor, London School of Hygiene and
Tropical Medicine
Keppel Street
London, UK

Trudie Roberts
Professor of Medical Education and
Director
Medical Education Unit
Worsley Building
University of Leeds
Leeds, UK

James E. Sabin
Director, Ethics Program, Harvard Pilgrim
Health Care
Clinical Professor, Departments of

Population Medicine and Psychiatry
Harvard Medical School
Boston, MA
USA

Norman Sartorius
Professor, Department of Psychiatry
University of Geneva
Geneva, Switzerland

Donna J. Schmutzler
Department of Health Services
Management
College of Public Health
University of Kentucky
Lexington, KY
USA

Zeryab Setna
Medical Education Unit
Worsley Building
University of Leeds
Leeds, UK

Bruce Singh
Professor, Department of Psychiatry
The University of Melbourne
Royal Melbourne Hospital
Victoria, Australia

John A. Talbott
Clinical Professor of Psychiatry
University of Maryland
Baltimore, MD
USA

Allan Tasman
Professor and Chairman
Department of Psychiatry and Behavioral
Sciences
University of Louisville School of
Medicine
Louisville, KY
USA

Jill Thistlethwaite
Director of the Institute of Clinical
Education (ICE)

Professor of Clinical Education and
Research
General Practitioner
University of Warwick
Coventry, UK

Kathy M. Vincent
Associate Professor and Vice Chair for
Education
Department of Psychiatry and Behavioral
Sciences
University of Louisville

Louisville, KY
USA

Sidney Weissman
Professor of Clinical Psychiatry
Department of Psychiatry and Behavioral
Science
Feinberg School of Medicine
Northwestern University
Chicago, IL
USA

Preface

Being a professional and behaving like one is about delivering services to an appropriately high standard, with a technical and scientific knowledge base, the skills learnt to deliver care and altruism as part of the professional responsibilities. The core values of a professional date back centuries and are embedded in moral links, trust, benevolence, courage, compassion and confidence, leading to truthfulness in professional relationships with patients and carers and with peers. Practical wisdom in medicine focuses on primacy of patient welfare and care. Learning about professionalism can start at an early stage as part of the undergraduate curriculum and can then be continued by learning through apprenticeship and mentoring at postgraduate level. Commitment to the highest possible standards of the profession and integrity are cornerstones of professionalism. Experts use patterns of work, recognition and training, whereas professionals go beyond being simple experts. Primacy of patient welfare, technical scientific knowledge and altruism are some of the core components of professionalism. It is inevitable that standards of patient welfare remain paramount, whereas scientific knowledge will continue to evolve and change. Altruism and its definitions change according to the society and healthcare system within which the professional practises. Definitions of healing also change as societies progress, but the role of the doctor as a healer dates back to antiquity.

In this volume, we bring together a group of international authors who for a number of years have been particularly interested in the field of medical professionalism. This volume is aimed at medical and psychiatric professionals for whom professionalism and expertise raise important issues. Lay readers and other professionals will find this book of value in understanding what medical and psychiatric professionalism is about and its components. We provide international comparisons, but it is clear that there are common strands, ethics and values running through medical professionalism, irrespective of the healthcare system in which practitioners work. This in itself is heartening as it indicates that it is the primacy of patient welfare which remains paramount. Transparency in treatment, honesty and probity are the watchwords. Modern medical ethics will continue to evolve whenever society's values, attitudes and beliefs change, but ethics remain important.

In addition, attaining expertise within the profession is significant, but an expert is not always a professional. The challenge for medical professionalism as a whole and for psychiatry in particular is to redefine its core values as a profession, and we hope that this volume will provide a useful focus.

We are grateful to our contributors, who have provided excellent overviews on time, in spite of their busy schedules. Thanks are also due to Richard Marley and his team at Cambridge University Press. For Andrea Livingstone and her major contribution, thanks alone are not sufficient. We are grateful.

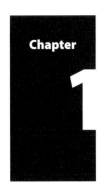

Chapter 1

Introduction
Experts and expertise

Dinesh Bhugra and Amit Malik

Experts in any field develop their expertise using both their training and experience. One of the key essentials of professionalism is embedded in the nature of the expertise of the profession. Underlying these attributes is the personality of the individual. Not every individual is good at everything, but all individuals have some skills which can lead to them becoming experts. The relationship between professionalism and expertise needs to be revisited, as not all professionals are experts and not all experts are necessarily professionals. The so-called oldest profession in the world is not necessarily related to level of expertise. Other professions, such as medicine, education and law, have different levels of expertise, depending upon a number of factors. The key to understanding professionalism is on two levels: first, what constitutes professionalism, and second, what gaps might highlight what a professional lacks, thus looking at expertise and professionalism both positively and negatively.

Experts are said to reach a level of skills where they can think clearly and rapidly and come to a quick and correct decision. Training to become an expert requires the acquisition of a number of skills. Skills are also linked with aptitude and attitude. Although skills can be learnt, aptitude and attitude may well be innate. The question often asked is whether experts, like good leaders, are born or made. The truth, as ever, is somewhere in the middle, indicating that skills can be learnt and practised, and that one can become proficient in them, but others are innate. The attitudes and components of professionalism are fluid and dynamic and change depending upon the circumstances and needs of society. Professionalism is defined as a socially sanctioned activity whose primary object is the wellbeing of others above the professional's personal gain (Racey 1990). Medicine, law and the ministry are the earliest examples of professionalism. Racey (1990) defines the virtues of a profession as moral links, fidelity to trust, benevolence, intellectual honesty, courage, compassion and truthfulness. The central virtue is said to be practical wisdom which unites moral and intellectual virtues. A considerable amount of learning is by practice, and best practice sometimes is to follow good role models. Embedded within this learning process are the components of skills and knowledge, which lead to personal and professional development. Expertise therefore takes on a new meaning. In craft specialties within medicine, repeated procedures allow individuals to gather experience and expertise. In art specialties such as psychiatry, clinical experience allows for professional development to occur in a different but distinct manner. Within the context of both professionalism and expertise, raising awareness of ethics and values through this learning experience is helpful in understanding subtle issues in an ever-changing complex world.

Professionalism in Mental Healthcare: Experts, Expertise and Expectations, ed. Dinesh Bhugra and Amit Malik. Published by Cambridge University Press. © Cambridge University Press 2011.

Professionalism is a large body of behaviour and beliefs which guide morally grounded physicians in their interactions with patients, their carers and families, other professionals and society at large (Page 2006). It is obvious that personal values such as greed, misrepresentation, abuse of power, breaches of confidentiality and exploitation of the vulnerable patient are totally unacceptable, and there is no justification for any of these behaviours. Physicians are also in danger of forfeiting a sizable portion of their status by ignoring patients' stories of their illnesses (Latham 2002).

Influential values in professionalism include professional autonomy and regulatory autonomy, patient autonomy, consumer sovereignty, patient advocacy, access to care and assurance of quality care (Preister 1992). These essential values are fundamental to the delivery of patient care, where the patient is at the pinnacle of the therapeutic interaction with high quality and efficiency. Instrumental values for the physician include personal responsibility, social solidarity, social advocacy, provider autonomy, consumer sovereignty and personal security. Preister (1992) goes on to define a new generation of essential values including access to care, efficiency and respect for patients. Specifically within mental healthcare, of these, access to care has to be both geographical and emotional access to services. Emotional access in psychiatry means that the services are not seen as stigmatizing and controlling.

As professionals, psychiatrists are experts not only in treating mental illness, but also in managing mental health problems associated with physical conditions and dealing with public mental health. This expertise is related to their roles as clinicians, researchers, teachers, managers and team players, in addition to their professional role as an advocate for their patients and their carers. One of the key skills embedded within this professional role is that of a good communicator. In the core therapeutic relationship, the professional must focus on the patient and the impact the patient's psychopathology is having on their social and personal functioning, exploring both the disease and the illness process with the patient (for a distinction between the two, see Eisenberg 1977). In any therapeutic encounter, an expert will explore the various dimensions that the illness causes for the patient, such as explanation, consequence, fears. The clinician must make every attempt to understand the whole person within the context of their society and culture. This is where the impact of social factors on illness must be explored thoroughly. In understanding the experiences, explanations and expressions of illness from the patient, the expert can engage with the patient, find common ground to explore, agree on goals of treatment and management plans and then keep these under review in regular discussions with the patient. The expert has to deal with the ambiguity of mental illness and also contain the anxiety not only of the patients and their carers but also of the team. These skills do not often come easily, but they can be learnt. Through a sense of vocation, compassion and awareness of the self and others, the expert can manage both simple and complex problems. *Good Psychiatric Practice* (RCPsych 2009) lists the attributes of a good psychiatrist, including providing good clinical care, a trusting relationship, confidentiality, teamwork, teaching and training and clinical governance, among other skills. Critical self-awareness and awareness of issues related to gender, ethnicity and culture, and the legal aspects of psychiatry, are also part of being a good clinician and a good psychiatrist. Therapeutic relationships with patients will produce transference and counter-transference, of which the psychiatrist needs to be aware and also work through in order to foster the clinical relationship.

Professionalism allows an individual not only to meet the standards set by others, but also to set standards for themselves. Under these circumstances, self-regulation takes on a different meaning in that, rather than the profession regulating itself, the individual takes on the responsibility of ensuring that they keep up-to-date and are fully aware of the nuances of clinical practice. This is not always easy. McNair (2005) points out that barriers in developing and maintaining professionalism include arrogance, abuse of power, lack of conscientiousness, conflicts of interest and uni-professionalism (pursuit of a goal for a single discipline to the exclusion of others). The development of professionalism must incorporate core areas of the framework of teaching – values, ethics, knowledge, skills for the process of learning and application (see Diaz 2006). Elcin *et al.* (2006) taught a course on professional identity to medical students and were able to show positive changes in all seven domains: the 'meaning' of being a doctor, expectations of professional identity, patient expectations of their doctors, professional limits of medical students, reactions of patients towards illness and death, reactions of physicians and situations faced in relation to patients. The study shows that attitudes and professional attributes can be changed.

In addition to other professional attributes of experts, knowledge of law, amongst other domains, needs to be looked at as a component of expert decision-making. Climo (1984) notes that in public mental hospitals, doctors must take into account what ordinary, well-meaning and responsible citizens might consider the right thing to do, above the guiding principles of either medicine or law. Under these circumstances, Climo (1984) suggests that the physician must ask two questions: first, what issues need to be resolved, a matter on which the staff should be able to advise; and second, what judgement is defensible if public accountability is demanded. Psychiatric decisions are often scrutinized by the legal system, especially in the context of risk assessment and management. Burstajn *et al.* (1984) point out that decision-making under these circumstances must look at the magnitude of the risk and the values or importance of that which is exposed to risk. A physician's acts must be measured against what other physicians would have done in similar circumstances. Burstajn *et al.* (1984) observe that these acts can founder on the inconsistency of medical knowledge, among other factors. In any analysis, personality and emotional, cognitive and philosophical factors must be taken into account. In collating a theory of clinical expertise, Kassirer *et al.* (1982) describe decision-making using protocols and protocol analysis. They note that physicians must learn thousands of configurations of findings in order to perform as experts. Citing the example of professional chess players who need over 50 000 configurations, these authors argue that talking about the problem changes the decision-making process. Therefore, turning a professional into an expert may require focusing on a different range of competencies. As stated before, not all experts are necessarily professionals, and neither are all professionals experts. The relationship between the two depends upon training and experience. Balint training in groups has been shown to be effective in developing insight into self by the trainees (Adams *et al.* 2006). Developing the students' professional self through the internalization of the values and virtues of medicine as a calling (vocation) and discipline requires a number of value orientations (Hafferty 2006). Personal reflection and self-awareness play an important part in becoming a professional and an expert.

Areas of expertise in psychiatry include culture; the ability to understand, co-ordinate and work co-operatively to provide comprehensive mental healthcare; the ability to understand ethical practice; and effective communication and education (Talbott and Mallott 2006). The concordance between professionalism and expertise needs to be emphasized further. Humanism in professionalism and in being an expert includes caring (defined as being concerned or interested in providing needed assistance or watchful supervision) and compassion (deep awareness of the suffering of another coupled with the will to relieve it) (Stern 2004).

Expertise also raises certain expectations from patients, their carers, families and society at large. Such expertise relies on experience gained by managing cases and working with patients. Expertise can be lost through external factors such as changing circumstances or context of clinical practice. It can also be lost as a result of internal or personal factors, e.g. addiction or illness. Gaining expertise is the first step, but retaining it is a major challenge.

The psychiatrist will need to be both an expert and a professional. Skills, knowledge, experience and the world view will all contribute towards this. Such attributes can be gained using different strategies, and the individual's development requires investment and resources.

O'Connor (2005) indicates that clinical practice guidelines articulate clear goals of care and enumerate potentially beneficial therapeutic approaches, which may reduce variations in care. O'Connor (2005) suggests that clinical practice guidelines are variably flawed in terms of conflict of interest, endorsement of newer interventions (which may be unproven) and a focus on a single condition. However, clinical practice guidelines are often difficult to employ in managing co-morbid conditions. Inevitably, all 'evidence-based' recommendations are not of equal clinical benefit to a patient. There need to be additional safeguards, such as looking at gender, age, costs, patient expectations and other factors, as noted by O'Connor (2005). Tinetti *et al.* (2004) point out other pitfalls associated with disease-specific guidelines for patients with multiple conditions. They suggest that medicine-related evidence which underlies the treatment guidelines only addresses the short-term disease-specific benefits of individual medications. They argue that the benefit/harm ratio, patient preferences and types of benefits from various combinations also need to be borne in mind. An awareness of the guidelines, their utility implications and their pitfalls all form part of the expert's portfolio. Ericsson (2004) states that individuals need experience to become professionals but extensive experience does not necessarily make people experts, and also notes that the limits of attainment of expertise are determined by one's basic endowments, such as one's innate and functional abilities, and mental capacities. Deliberate practice is at the heart of both expertise and professionalism. Whereas initial expertise is related to engagement in deliberate practice, continued deliberate practice is essential for maintaining professional performance (Ericsson 2004). It takes up to 10 years of professional development to become an expert. Ericsson (2004) stresses that the principal difference between the acquisition of everyday skills and professional development is related to differences in timescale. Motivation plays an important role, and the sense of purpose and vocation could be linked with motivation.

Expert performers have to be trained to such a level that they can reproduce their superior performance under representative conditions in everyday life whenever it is required during competition and training (Ericsson 2004). According to Ericsson (2004), acquisition of expertise occurs across different domains and at different paces, and deliberate practice is designed to improve specific aspects of performance in such a way that all the changes can be integrated into representative performance. Expert performance in medicine relies on long periods of training and a long time for knowledge and continued professional development. Steps in learning depend upon establishing tasks which define the domains and then learning and practising such tasks to build on existing skills. Ericsson *et al.* (1993) define deliberate practice as highly structured activity aiming to improve performance, to overcome weakness and carefully monitor performance. Of course, deliberate practice requires time, energy and motivation. Introduction to an activity ends with the start of the instruction and deliberate practice followed by extended periods of preparation and full-time commitment. Bloom (1985) goes on to emphasize that external support is required in all these stages and, as an expert, they go beyond the knowledge of teachers to make major innovative contributions to their domain. Constraints which may influence the development of expertise include poor resources and lack of interest and effort, all of which may occur singly or in combination. As Ericsson *et al.* (1993) note, expert performance is qualitatively different from normal performance, though there may be some commonalities and some differences in level and style. The relationship between training, expertise and professionalism needs to be explored further.

References

Adams K E, O'Reilly M, Romm J, James K (2006). Effect of Balint training on resident professionalism. *American Journal of Obstetrics & Gynecology* **195**, 431–437.

Bloom B S (1985). Generalizations about talent development. In B S Bloom (ed.) *Developing Talent in Young People*. New York: Ballantine, pp. 507–549.

Burstajn H, Hamm R M, Gutheil T G, Brodsky A (1984). The decision analytic approach to medical malpractice law. *Medical Decision Making* **4**, 401–414.

Climo L H (1984). Some thorny medical judgements and their outcomes: the view from the public mental hospital. *Medical Decision Making* **4**, 415–424.

Diaz A (2006). Can you advocate healthcare students in interprofessionalism. *Clinical Teacher* **3**, 4–6.

Eisenberg L (1977). Disease and illness: distinction between professional and popular ideas of sickness. *Culture Medicine and Psychiatry* **1**, 9–23.

Elcin M, Odabasi O, Gokler B, Sayek I, Akova M, Kiper N (2006). Developing and evaluating professionalism. *Medical Teacher* **28**, 36–39.

Ericsson K A (2004). Deliberate practice and the acquisition and maintenance of expert performance in medicine and related domains. *Academic Medicine* **79**, Suppl S1–S12.

Ericsson K A, Krampe R T, Tech-Römer C (1993). The role of deliberate practice in the acquisition of expert performance. *Psychological Review* **100**, 363–406.

Hafferty F W (2006). Professionalism – the new wave. *New England Journal of Medicine* **355**, 2151–2152.

Kassirer J P, Kuipers B J, Gorry G A (1982). Towards a theory of clinical expertise. *American Journal of Medicine* **73**, 251–259.

Latham S R (2002). Medical professionalism. *Mt Sinai Journal of Medicine* **69**, 363–369.

McNair R P (2005). The case for educating healthcare students in professionalism on the core content of interprofessional education. *Medical Education* **39**, 456–464.

O'Connor P J (2005). Adding value to evidence based clinical guidelines. *Journal of the American Medical Association* **294**, 741–743.

Page D W (2006). Professionalism and team care in the clinical setting. *Clinical Anatomy* **19**, 468–472.

Preister R (1992). A values framework for health system reform. *Health Affairs* **11**, 84–107.

Racey J (1990). Professionalism: sane and insane. *Journal of Clinical Psychiatry* **51**, 138–140.

Royal College of Psychiatrists (2009). *Good Psychiatric Practice* (3rd edn). London: RCPysch Press.

Stern D T (2004). *Measuring Medical Professionalism*. New York: Oxford University Press.

Talbott J M, Mallott D B (2006). Professionalism, medical humanism and clinical bioethics: the new wave – does psychiatry have a role? *Journal of Psychiatric Practice* **12**, 384–390.

Tinetti M E, Bogardus S T, Agostini J V (2004). Potential pitfalls of disease-specific guidelines for patients with multiple conditions. *New England Journal of Medicine* **351**, 2870–2874.

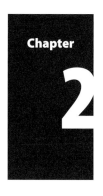

Chapter

2

Globalization

Norman Sartorius

Editors' introduction

In an increasingly shrinking world, the contacts between cultures and communities are becoming closer. The economic and social impact of the process of globalization can be understood at several levels – that of the individual, the family, culture, society, etc. – and the different systems get influenced at different speeds. For example, the economic system changes and responds to the needs of globalization at a faster pace in comparison with the political systems. With globalization, two additional factors – urbanization and industrialization – may come into play, contributing to additional social stresses. Rapid transition from agrarian societies with perhaps more traditional attitudes and values to industrialized societies competing in the international market-place will change attitudes, beliefs and behaviours. Changes in economic patterns may further add to increasing social disparity and poverty, perhaps in the short run. The impact of two cultures coming into contact with each other will affect the way each one looks at professionalism. Professional standards in one country are therefore likely to affect how services are delivered and social expectations evolve within others. Globalization also encourages trained professionals from low- and middle-income countries to rich countries.

Sartorius observes that the introduction of a free market economy into healthcare systems had led to the destruction of previously well-established primary care systems. It is likely that public mental health will be seen to be less important in largely private healthcare systems. Changes in the middle class, with expansions in numbers and altered expectations, will influence changes at multiple levels. Commoditification of healthcare provides a further sense of alienation among the poor. Globalization also reduces social capital, which has previously promoted interdependence, survival and mutual trust. Migration, changing relations between countries and socio-demographic changes will influence training and standards of expertise. Changes in value systems are likely to occur. Clinicians and trainers need to be aware of the impact (both overt and covert) of globalization.

Introduction

Globalization was experienced as a possible beautiful dream in the early 1960s. After the horrors of the Second World War and the momentous developments – such as decolonization – that followed it, nothing seemed more attractive than living in a world with open borders and with a free circulation of ideas, wares, people, objects of art and culture. The osmosis

Professionalism in Mental Healthcare: Experts, Expertise and Expectations, ed. Dinesh Bhugra and Amit Malik. Published by Cambridge University Press. © Cambridge University Press 2011.

of ideologies that would lessen the strengths of reasons for conflicts in the future appeared possible.

As time went on, however, the dark side of globalization gained the upper hand. The borders were open within groups of countries, not across the world. The ideologies and value systems of the economically most powerful were imposed on those less fortunate. The free circulation of ideas was replaced by a mono-directional flow of soap operas and news about events in a small number of countries. The productivity of agriculture and industry continued to grow in the First World, suppressing the economic and industrial development in the developing countries.

This chapter will examine some of the components of globalization which, in recent years, became somewhat more useful to all, possibly because of the realization that a variety of the world's problems can only be resolved jointly, by all countries facing the world's challenges together.

Decivilization

Civilization can be measured by the amount of attention that a society pays to its feeble members – children, the elderly, the disabled and others who need support in order to live a life of acceptable quality or to survive (Sartorius 2009a). An indicator of the state of civilization might be a comparison of the gross national product and child mortality or the purchasing power of the retirement pension of the elderly in comparison with the purchasing power of those employed. Accessibility and quality of healthcare to the majority of the population could also be used to assess how civilized a society has become.

Recent years have unfortunately shown that some of the countries that had previously succeeded in reducing child mortality – such as most of the countries of Eastern Europe and of the Community of Independent States assembling previous parts of the USSR – are no longer maintaining their respectably low level reached in the years before and after the Second World War. In other countries that are achieving prodigious economic growth, the level of support for public health measures and in particular the support for those disabled – not infrequently by consequences of unprotected labour – are remaining low or non-existent. The introduction of market economy in a country such as Mongolia (which had previously established a well-functioning primary healthcare system) led to the development of private healthcare facilities and a significant weakening of the peripheral health services. In other countries, rapid industrial development led to an increase in environmental pollution, with consequent health problems and none or almost no improvement of coverage by healthcare of the non-employed part of the population. What is worse is that much of the environmental deterioration happens in countries which have a poorly developed health service. Indeed, of the seven most polluted sites in the world, five are in developing countries (Mexico City, Mexico: air pollution; Niger Delta, Nigeria: crude oil pollution; Dhaka, Bangladesh: waste water pollution; Linfen, China: coal mining and air pollution; Mumbai, India: air, water and waste pollution), and two are in Eastern Europe (Norilsk, Russia: heavy metal and air pollution; Chernobyl, Ukraine: radioactive pollution).[1]

---

[1] Source: www.groundreport.com, Blacksmith Institute, Green Cross International, cited in China Post, 8 November 2009.

The changes of the middle class

The changes of the middle class have had a profound impact on healthcare and on the social fabric of societies. The size of the middle class in developing countries has grown and led to a variety of consequences. Although the middle-class proportion of the population in developing countries is still small, the total numbers of middle-class citizens became very large. Thus, India has more middle-class citizens than the United States, and in Africa there are by the latest counts some 80 000 millionaires (Sartorius 2009b). Moreover, in many Third World countries, 10 to 15% of the population have incomes that are comparable to those in the Western European countries. This, of course, does not mean that the numbers of poor people became smaller; they have also grown, although in terms of percentage they have somewhat diminished.

A large number of people with a middle-class status and income meant that the countries in which they live became interesting markets for both home and foreign industry. This is also true for the health industry, and in many developing countries private healthcare (and private mental healthcare) has grown in size and in quality. Middle-class citizens are no longer interested in or relying on primary healthcare services that the governments in most of the Third World countries tried to build up. Primary healthcare remained important for the poorer portion of the population, which grows disenchanted with it, not least also because they can see that their more fortunate brothers are benefiting from much better care in the same country.

The situation is worsened even further by the fact that the 'brain drain' that was previously due mainly to emigration to other, richer countries has now become stronger for two reasons: first, because some of the highly developed countries such as the UK actively encouraged 'brain drain' by offering attractive conditions of work to immigrant experts; and second, because the private healthcare system siphoned out many of the best young graduates, who flocked to private institutions rather than accepting to serve with a lower salary and worse working conditions in government services.

The middle class did not change only in the developing world. In many industrialized countries the middle class has diminished in size and influence. The middle class was at all times the protector of the morale it created: as it became weaker, so did adherence to moral rules and values, leading to uncertainty and dissatisfaction among the population and to the worsening of indicators of social malaise and disruption such as the increase in violence (e.g. in schools), suicide and criminality.

Commoditification

Commoditification is a new word indicating the gradual conversion of all interactions and activity into economic terms. Thus, healthcare is handled as a commodity in a similar way to sugar, cotton or other commodities. The consequent emphasis on reducing the cost of healthcare in order to make it cost-effective has unfortunately often been accompanied by a worsening of the quality of healthcare. The savings on health calculated year by year sound good to the decision-makers, who often do not see or do not want to remember the fact that at a later date these savings will result in dangerous consequences. The part of the healthcare budget that was to be used for preventive activities has been diminished in most countries. Those who are not likely to fully recover from their ailments are less likely to receive good care. Return to employment of those who have received treatment is often the main criterion of effectiveness, such that the treatment of diseases likely to result in some form of long-lasting impairment (e.g. severe mental illness) receives very little attention. Government regulations (or regulations of insurance companies and HMOs), for example, have replaced the physician's choice of medications, which are often selected on the basis of their low cost rather than on the basis of a judicious consideration of all of their characteristics, including their side effects and the patients' experience.

Commoditification of the health system contributes to the dissatisfaction of the population with their healthcare and to a renewed growth of alternative medicine, which is experienced as being less dehumanized than the exclusively economically minded health system that is supposedly based on scientific evidence. The magic wand of traditional and alternative medicine had been torn in the late decades of the twentieth century, but it has been gaining new strength in recent years, often to the detriment of the health of those who sought healthcare outside of the health system, which they experienced as disagreeable and excessively commercialized.

Reduction of the social capital

The capital of a society is composed of three elements: the economic capital, including all material goods that a society possesses; the human capital, referring to the productivity of a society; and the social capital, equal to the sum of actions that citizens do to help each other (Sartorius 2003). One of the chief measures of social capital is the trust that members of society have in each other, and one of the main characteristics of societies with high levels of social capital is the interdependence of its members. Social capital is often the main protector of survival in societies with little economic capital and with poor productivity.[2] The increase in the economic capital of a society – through input of material resources (e.g. donations from other countries or of the discovery of natural resources) or through a growth of human capital – usually decreases the social capital. The material wealth makes members of society replace support that they owe to others by money. In the beginning this practice hides the disappearance of social capital; soon, however, the purchase of social support (e.g. domestic help) becomes too expensive, and a number of tasks that are necessary for the survival of well-functioning societies remain undone. The increase in the cost of healthcare seen and lamented in most developed countries is to a large extent due to the fact that family members are no longer able or willing to care for their mentally or physically impaired members. In the developing countries the notion that families are strong and will remain strong is still an article of faith for most decision-makers; the trend of decreasing family size and the failure of healthcare models relying on continuing strong support of extended families, which can be seen in some of the countries that have succeeded in speeding up their economic growth, are unfortunately not influencing this notion.

Social capital is decreasing in most societies, particularly in those that have experienced the fastest economic growth and achieved some prosperity. The consequences of this change for healthcare and for other pursuits that, to a large extent, depend on high levels of social capital (e.g. survival of the elderly with functional impairments) are vast and unpleasant.

---

[2] The economic miracle of Japan's recovery and growth after the Second World War was in part due to the emphasis on *amae*, interdependence highly regarded by traditional Japanese culture.

Migration and population movements

The mobility of individuals and populations is increasing in most parts of the world. Even in countries in which the proportion of persons who migrate is stagnant or decreasing, the number of migrants is larger than ever before. Migration does not stop at the move of people from one place to another. Migrants bring their systems of values with them and these are sometimes incompatible with their hosts' cultures. They also bring their diseases or the ways in which diseases express themselves in other parts of the world. In travel, the latter often change and become different from the expressions of the disease in the home and in the host countries, leaving the health workers of both countries baffled and uncertain about the treatment and about other measures they should undertake.

Migration across borders is more visible and its effects are observed with more attention than migration within borders. A huge proportion of the population, particularly in developing countries, is moving to cities, contributing to the rapid urbanization of the planet. The most urbanized country in the world – Argentina, with more than four fifths of its population living in cities – was until recently a country whose strength and population were outside of urban areas. Countries such as China had the vast majority of its population living in rural areas until very recently; now, nearly half of its citizens have moved to towns. Urban populations require a system of healthcare that is different from that serving well in rural areas; while this fact is recognized by many, there is still no well-articulated generally accepted strategy of urban healthcare. The operational prescriptions of primary healthcare that the World Health Organization has been promoting over the past 40 years are appropriate for use in rural areas of the world, but they do not have their counterpart in a primary healthcare strategy for use in urban areas (Sartorius 1998).

The technological revolution

The technological revolution and in particular the amazing advances of the technology of information management have also contributed to the changes of societies. The modern media bring the same information about events – catastrophic and other – into the vast majority of households worldwide. The Internet opens the doors to a world of information about all possible subjects including diseases and their management. Surgical operations that could previously be seen only in science fiction movies are often performed in provincial medical centres. The new and modern 'exoskeleton' of humans – allowing a single worker operating a crane to move hundreds of tons of material and making it possible to fly thousands of miles in metal boxes called aeroplanes – makes incredibly complex and difficult feats normal and expected.

Unfortunately, however, the new technology has not sufficiently reduced the distance between the rich and the poor: the new apparatus is not evenly available or used by all. The per capita number of personal computers, for example, is much higher in the developed than in the non-industrialized countries. Those who can afford to purchase computers also have access to training in their use. Those who are well off can use fast and safe vehicles of transport which are much more costly than those old, dangerous and slow ones that have to be used by poorer people. The distance between the poor and uneducated and those who have education and resources to use the new technology is growing. The disadvantages of the poor and the advantages of those who are better off are accumulating and lead to an increase in inequity and consequent malaise and social disruption.

Another, unexpected consequence of the introduction of information technology into everyday life is increasingly apparent in many countries and particularly among those of younger age. The possibility of communicating with others by machines has reduced the use of social and interpersonal skills to the point that many are forgotten. An increasing number of studies from many countries report that a significant number of young people remain restricted to electronic communication with others or with the anonymous World Wide Web; the contacts with their parents are reduced to a minimum and often begin and end at accepting the food being offered. Direct social contacts with others have ceased.[3] Food and other necessities are ordered by telephone. The contacts with family members are restricted to electronic communication. Young people will make suicide pacts with others whom they have never seen (and with whom they have only Internet links) and then kill themselves at a set time that they have selected together. Friends are not invited to come to one's home to share food and talk any longer. Telling jokes has become an almost extinct skill since television brought the world's best comic actors into everyone's home. Communication among colleagues having offices next to each other is done by email. Courses for young professionals now have to include the learning of skills which in previous times were an essential part of the education at home, living with siblings and various family members. The developing countries are somewhat better off in this respect; however, it is clearly probable that similar trends will also become apparent in those lands at present still largely dependent on interpersonal and emotional links and communication. The recent estimate that at least half of the population of Africa now has mobile phones is an indicator of the magnitude and speed of this change.

Obsolescence of social service strategies

Several of the strategies of social service that were developed in the twentieth century have become obsolete. They are still taught in schools of health and by other social service personnel, still used as a basis for governmental policies and budgeting, still hailed as being the best way to a glorious future. Thus, for example, strategies of healthcare promote community healthcare and the reliance on the community in the organization of preventive interventions; however, in most countries of the world, communities in the sense in which they were functioning at the time when community care strategies were designed are disappearing. The proportion of the populations living in rural areas is constantly diminishing, and urban populations do not form communities which are geographically defined and in which people not only know one another but also have long-standing links, often based on mutual help over many generations.

The same health policy documents that promote reliance on community care also omit any mention of private healthcare systems, even in countries in which the majority of the population has to rely on it. The private sector is not only assuming an increasing importance and responding to much of the service needs, it has also massively invaded education and drains a significant proportion of health personnel. The notion that policies for healthcare can omit the mention of the private sector is probably a remnant of the situation after the Second World War, when there was a general tendency to consider governments as the

---

[3] A syndrome of social withdrawal – the Hikikomori syndrome, as this behavioural style has been labelled – has struck an estimated 1 million people in Japan. Reports from other countries indicate that the problem is not exclusively Japanese but may be a real menace to all the world's countries.

main providers for all citizens. This has indeed happened in all Eastern European countries and in many of the other countries of Europe, as well as in Canada and elsewhere. Some of the developing countries have moved in the same direction and provided essential, minimal healthcare to all of the population. In many more countries, however, the government's role in providing care was minimal, sometimes reaching only a minute proportion of the population employed in the civil services. The withdrawal of governments from the role of provider of care has now become a general trend, yet policies and officially proclaimed plans for social services seem to be oblivious of this trend.

Even the eight Millennium Development Goals, formulated much later, suffer from the allegiance to principles and ideas that were almost obsolete when the goals were formulated and became even more obsolete over time. Thus, the goal directed to disease control specifies 'HIV/AIDS, malaria and other diseases,' but of all the other diseases tuberculosis is the only one that gets attention. There is no doubt that HIV/AIDS, malaria and tuberculosis deserve attention and produce a great deal of disability and misery, but they are by far not the only disorders that a Millennium Goal of disease control should specify. Other diseases that are not mentioned among the targets produce an incomparably larger burden of disability and will have to be tackled if countries are to develop their full socio-economic potential.

Changing relations between countries

Despite the remarkable economic progress achieved in some of the developing countries, the gap between the majority of poor countries and the rich ones is still increasing. This difference is, however, not evenly distributed among the different pursuits of society. While the life of poor people is as miserable as – or worse than – before, the numbers of academically active people, for example, have grown in many developing countries, and their scientific excellence gives much hope for the growth of locally relevant knowledge and for major contributions to science in general from the Third World. This development is not only of scientific significance: it has also implications for the relationships between experts in different countries. In the past, the experts from highly developed countries enjoyed huge authority, and their pronouncements were nearly always considered as having more weight than anything that was said by the local scientists or practitioners. This is no longer so, and scientists and experts from both industrialized and developing countries have to learn a new language and a new style of behaviour appropriate for partnership among equals.

At present, this is not happening in all instances. Arrogance and disrespect can still be the main obstacle to the development of collaborative programmes of research and training that would not only make the acquisition of knowledge faster, but could also open new vistas, an almost normal by-product of equitable international collaboration. Differences of researchers' income between countries can also be an obstacle to the development of equitable collaboration, in that researchers in poorer countries can often be engaged in research that is not a priority for their country nor for their academic institution but pays well or allows the purchase of apparatus and travel to other lands.

Socio-demographic changes

Socio-demographic changes – the increase in the absolute and relative numbers of the elderly, the changing roles of women, the growing rates of divorce and the decrease in birth rate in most countries (with the exception of the Middle East and African countries with predominantly Muslim populations) – are undoubtedly influenced by globalization, which is proposing or imposing role models that modern communication technology brings to all corners of the Earth. Many societies have managed to survive because they adopted lifestyles that were useful for the survival of the group, albeit not always agreeable to its members. Globalization has disrupted these lifestyles, mainly by showing that elsewhere people live differently and seem to be flourishing. Yet, these new ways – clearly logical and attractive as they may be for the individual – are not helping societies to grow and develop because they are introduced far too rapidly without preparation, often in disharmony with the existing culture and in contradiction with the principles that underlie the fabric of society. Even the provision of general education, for example, without proper training of teachers and adequate social arrangements, can result in considerable misery and ruined lives of those whom failure in school will mark as being slower to learn than their peers and therefore labelled as mentally retarded who should be excluded from society. Such a by-product of the efforts to reach the Millennium Goal of general education is not trivial. Estimates from a variety of countries show that mild forms of intellectual disability reach 4 to 5% of the general population.

The changing role of women has a variety of consequences. In traditional societies, women are those who transmit culture, care for the sick and disabled members of the family, bring up children and often also contribute to the income of the family by working part-time outside the house. Once fully employed outside their home they usually have to continue with their traditional duties but do them less well because there are limits to what a person can do in the course of a day. The break in the transmission of culture and the imperfect rearing of children are consequences that will become visible in the future; the interruption of care for the elderly and disabled is reflected much sooner in the increase in the cost of healthcare and in higher mortality of the infirm and the elderly. Governments and international organizations recognize the problem but do little to provide the resources that will allow employment of women while ensuring that the traditional contribution of women to society is maintained.

Importation of value systems

Globalization has been marked by the imposition of value systems from the more powerful, economically developed countries to the rest of the world. Many of the values that have been transmitted can support the growth and development of societies as well as the improvement of quality of life and its many constituents. Some of them, however, do not. These often sprang from the specific history, geographical position and challenges that the society had to face and faced successfully.

An example of such an imposed value is the striving to achieve independence of the individuals in a society, particularly after an illness. Fiercely promoted and embedded in a variety of contexts, it has reached countries in which the cultural tradition and survival of society did not rest on the independence of individuals composing the society but on their interdependence. Interdependence means a number of obligations for each of the members of the society, but it also means that the sources of help, when help is needed, are numerous. The acceptance of independence meant that the mutual protection and help resulting from interdependence – which was often the main source of strength of a community – vanished without being replaced by some of the structures that exist in the countries in which the notion of independence gathered strength. The 'fish brotherhoods' of the Inuits on Greenland were a striking example of interdependence: when one of them caught a fish, he was obliged to provide specified parts of it – a fin, or the head perhaps – to his 'fin brother' or his 'head brother'. The catch was thus divided among the 'brothers' and ensured that they survived even if they did not all have the same luck in catching the fish every time. To help the community, the government built a factory and purchased the fish that was caught, paying a fair price for it; the problem that was not foreseen was that the fishermen spent their money without sharing it, usually on alcohol or objects that were to their own liking. They have thus become more independent and could compete with each other, leaving those less able or less lucky to look after themselves in any way they could. The principles of independence and free competition were introduced and their introduction hailed as a sign of progress and liberation, although their acceptance led to the detriment of the group as a whole.

Sometimes the values were imported in the envelope of a religion that the colonizing power tried to impose on the population in the colony. Conversion to the new religion and the acceptance of its morality by some members of the society often resulted in intergenerational and other conflicts that damaged the unity of the group and reduced its capacity to survive and grow. Sometimes values are embedded in laws that are introduced or copied because in their place of origin they have been seen as highly progressive and useful. The insistence that there must be laws covering every aspect of life has unfortunately often led to the transmission of legislation that is not appropriate for the culture and socio-economic status of the country into which they were imported.

The predominance of the major languages of the colonizing powers of the past – English, French, Spanish and Russian – has the great advantage of making communication globally possible; unfortunately, however, the acceptance of a language also means that the values that are prevalent in the country of its origin will be imposed imperceptibly because they are contained in the choice of words and in their literal meaning.

Coda

This chapter addressed some of the issues related to globalization. It did not attempt to provide a comprehensive analysis of the phenomenon and of all its consequences; rather, it listed examples and notions that are relevant to the understanding of the impact that globalization has on all aspects of human life, including the functioning of health and other social services. Globalization is not likely to go away, although its many negative consequences and corruptions make it an anathema for significant parts of society. It has many positive aspects and carries a lot of promise for the development of human societies worldwide; the fulfilment of its promise and potential will require the efforts and patience of many, including also those who see only its negative features. The health professions have a major role to play in this respect, because of their leadership role in many societies and because the exercise of their profession depends on finding hidden strength in individuals and communities in disease and in distress.

References

Sartorius N (1998). Mental health needs of an urbanized planet. In D Goldberg, G Thornicroft (eds.) *Mental Health in our Future Cities*. London: Psychology Press Ltd, Taylor & Frances Group, pp. 5–13.

Sartorius N (2003). Social capital and mental health. In C R Soldatos (Guest Editor). Challenges in Contemporary Psychiatry. A Special Issue in Honour of Professor Costas N. Stefanis. *Current Opinion in Psychiatry* **16**(Suppl 2), 101–105.

Sartorius N (2009a). *Medicine in the Era of Decivilization*. The works of the Croatian Academy of Sciences and Arts, Number 504, Volume XXXIII Medical Sciences.

Sartorius N (2009b). *Pathways of Medicine*. Zagreb: Medicinska Naklada.

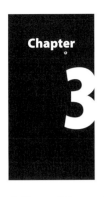

Chapter 3

The virtues and vices of professionalism

Jonathan Montgomery

Editors' introduction

Ethical and legal aspects related to medical professionalism and expertise are significant but are often ignored in training, at both undergraduate and postgraduate levels. However, in recent times this is beginning to change. Increasingly, experts are becoming aware that their expertise has to be earned, retained and developed within the social, legal, cultural and ethical constraints. Probity is one of the key components in medical professionalism. As psychiatrists are often seen as the agents of social control, it is inevitable that the legal framework will play an important role in clinical practice and in the delivery of psychiatric services. This is further complicated by risk assessment and risk management. In this chapter, Montgomery points out the altruistic service ethic in which the expertise of the professional was secured for society through (an implicit) contract with society. Changing social and economic circumstances and expectations mean that altruistic behaviour itself may need to be redefined. Of course professionalism and its values can be criticized as being self-serving, especially if self-regulation is included in the equation. Montgomery points out that with regard to medicine, the law takes to an extreme degree the role of expertise and peers, rather than simply employing external standards. Judges have thus far shied away from defining the standards expected of medical professionals. Montgomery asserts that the law has built on an image of medical professionalism a particular model of healthcare law that assumes and furthermore promotes the moral basis of medical practice. How does this moral basis fit into legal and medical paradigms? Legal decisions and judgements have highlighted both moral and technical bases for the professional role. The challenge for clinicians in these days of increasing guidelines and economic constraints is whether there remains such a thing as clinical freedom, if indeed there ever was. The role of the professional keeps evolving, and the challenge for the profession is to respond to social changes and expectations.

Introduction

Professionalism is a characteristic that can mean many different things. For some, it is the opposite of amateurism – demonstrating the systematic application of expertise in contrast to the blundering of a well-meaning but ill-equipped enthusiast. In this sense, the rise of professionalism is illustrated by the replacement of the Victorian gentleman's hobby by the modern career scientist. In a modern technologically driven society, to be a professional in this sense is usually a compliment. Other senses are less clearly positive. In some uses, the

Professionalism in Mental Healthcare: Experts, Expertise and Expectations, ed. Dinesh Bhugra and Amit Malik. Published by Cambridge University Press. © Cambridge University Press 2011.

adjective 'professional' captures the detachment required to replace the personal subjectivity of a merely sympathetic emotional reaction with an objective response based on empathy, evidence and careful deliberation. Here, 'professionalism' is (at least in part) a defence against the stresses arising from conflicts between the demands of a person's occupational role and their personal integrity – that is, the instinctive responses generated by their own identities and individual reactions to the circumstances in which their work places them. People are said to behave 'professionally' when they continue to perform their normal work roles despite personal provocation (such as threats of violence, blackmail or bribery) or emotional connections with their clients. While this is usually a positive sense of professionalism, and one that those who train professionals will applaud, it can also carry a hint of coldness and lack of a caring attitude that is not always welcomed by 'clients', who may find it dismissive and a source of frustration.

Moving beyond the attributes of individuals to groups, an even greater disparity of views can be seen. George Bernard Shaw famously described the professions as a 'conspiracy against the laity' but they have seen themselves rather differently. In 2005 a working party convened by the Royal College of Physicians, under the chairmanship of former health minister Baroness Julia Cumberlege, took extensive evidence on what professionalism meant to key health service personnel and to doctors at various stages in their careers (Royal College of Physicians 2005b). The working party drew up an explanation of the demands of modern professionalism based on the understanding that

Medicine is a vocation in which a doctor's knowledge, clinical skills, and judgement are put in the service of protecting and restoring human well-being. This purpose is realised through a partnership between patient and doctor, one based on mutual respect, individual responsibility, and appropriate accountability. (Royal College of Physicians 2005a:14)

This approach resonates with the classic work of the sociologist Talcott Parsons, who explained how the special position of professions in society was based on an altruistic service ethic in which the expertise of the professional was secured for society through a social contract that provided status and financial security without a direct link to financial reward, transaction by transaction (Parsons 1939). Breaching this social contract would put the continuation of professional services at risk.

Not all sociologists have been so sympathetic to the claims on which professional status is based. Terence Johnson has emphasized professionalism as a mechanism for protecting occupational power. He suggests that the principal characteristic of professions is their ability to dominate their clients and occupational competitors. Thus, professional 'producers' are able to define first the needs of consumers and then also the ways in which those needs will be met. This control is justified by reference to esoteric knowledge that ensures a distance is maintained between the competent expert professional and the ignorant lay client. Professional power is maintained by a process of mystification whereby the uncertainty of the relevant knowledge reinforces the incompetence of the lay client (Johnson 1972). Seen from such a perspective, traditional claims to professional self-regulation are seen as cynical strategies for the maintenance of power rather than the natural implications of professional expertise and altruistic values.

If this is what professionalism means, then it is difficult to defend it in the context of modern health services. This chapter explores what can be learnt about the nature of professionalism through the lens of the law. It shows how the law has been used to reinforce professional power and how the development of legal doctrine has been predicated on historical assumptions about professionals that may be of doubtful legitimacy and which need defending in contemporary terms. However, it is also contended that some of the themes that can be seen emerging within the domain of law contribute to the basis for a legitimate sense of professionalism.

Translating professionalism into law

English healthcare law has been heavily influenced by the concept of professionalism (Montgomery 1989), and it is possible to trace some of the less attractive characteristics to which Johnson drew attention. The law has generally reflected rather than overcome the power that medicine has exerted over other health professions (Montgomery 1992), and too often it has been little more than a tool for asserting independence and a weapon in the fight for exalted social status (Montgomery 1998). Where the law merely reinforces the social and economic structure of the division of health labour in this way, it offers few clues to how we should respond to claims for professionalism. However, in some areas its rationales are less reactive to power and more constitutive of a normative structure for professionalism. Here, we may stand to learn something more useful.

This can be explored in the law's approach to clinical negligence. The legal doctrine of negligence is used to determine when one person should pay compensation to another because they have not exercised due care, and their failure to do so caused harm to the 'victim' of the mishap. In ordinary circumstances, the judiciary determines what degree of care the law expects people to take, forming a view against the yardstick of 'reasonableness'. In cases of professional negligence, the position is slightly different; here the test incorporates aspects of prevailing practice from the profession in question. The test that is usually used was set out in an early informed consent case and is known as the *Bolam* test after the plaintiff in that case (Bolam v W Friern HMC 1957). Under that test

a doctor is not guilty of negligence if he has acted in accordance with a practice accepted as proper by a responsible body of medical men skilled in that particular art.

This test fixes the required standard of care not by reference to the judge's assessment of a reasonable balance of risk but by reference to peer review. Provided that a responsible body of the practitioner's peers accept that their practice was 'proper', then, even if the judge were minded to disagree, the practitioner would not be liable to pay compensation.

Thus far, this is essentially a matter for professionals in general. In the context of medicine, it is clear that the law takes to an extreme degree the incorporation of expertise into the law rather than judging its reasonableness by external standards. The high water mark of such judicial deference can be seen in the development of three glosses on this test that come close to excluding judicial scrutiny of medical practice. First, the fact that judges have concluded that it is not for them to choose between schools of professional thought, so that complying with one of them is sufficient to protect the doctor even where the issue is the cause of controversy within the profession (Maynard v West Midlands AHA RHA 1985). Second, it is now clear that even a small group of specialists can constitute a 'responsible body of opinion' (De Freitas v O'Brien 1995). Putting these two developments together, it can be seen that doctors are close to being immune from litigation provided that they comply with a basic level of medical practice.

Commentators, including senior judges (Scarman 1987), have long observed that this seems to enable doctors to police themselves, and some effort has been made to restrict the

Bolam principle to areas of technical expertise. However, this was roundly rejected by Lord Diplock, who, in the third gloss on *Bolam*, asserted that

The general duty is not subject to dissection into a number of component parts to which different criteria of what satisfies the duty of care apply, such as diagnosis, treatment, advice … no convincing reason has in my view been advanced before your Lordships that would justify treating the *Bolam* test as doing anything less than laying down a principle of English law that is comprehensive and applicable to every aspect of the duty of care owed by a doctor to his patient. (Sidaway v Bethlem RHG 1985)

The judges have begun to express some disquiet at the deference that this approach shows to medical professionalism (Woolf 2001), and there is evidence that expert witnesses are being pushed rather harder than had been the case on whether they really regard a practice as proper. The courts have asserted the right to assess the logical consistency of medical practice (Bolitho v City & Hackney HA 1997). However, there seems little evidence that judges have been prepared to take over the task of defining the standards expected of medical professionals (Montgomery 2000, 2003).

    The most satisfactory explanation for this approach seems to lie in the adoption by the judiciary of an understanding of professionalism that mirrors closely the self-image that was captured by the work of Talcott Parsons. The relevant judicial attitudes can be traced through a number of areas of law (Montgomery 1989). Concern has been expressed about the technical nature of medical issues, such that the law 'must take the standard of care and diligence of a surgeon from those who could alone from their expert knowledge inform them of it' (Mahon v Osborne 1939:557). Judges can be found to say that medical negligence is different to other types of negligence claim: 'A charge of professional negligence against a medical man was serious. … It affected his professional status and reputation.' (Lord Denning in Hucks v Cole 1960). One extract from the Court of Appeal displays particularly neatly the attitudes that were held:

If the unit had not been there, the plaintiff would probably have died. The doctors and nurses worked all kinds of hours to look after the baby. They safely brought it through the perilous shoals of its early life. For all that we know, they far surpassed on numerous occasions the standard of reasonable care. Yet it is said that for one lapse they (and not just their employers) are to be found to have committed a breach of duty. Nobody could criticise the mother for doing her best to secure her son's financial future. But has not the law taken a wrong turning if an action of this kind is to succeed? (Wilsher v Essex AHA 1986, per Mustill L J)

Lord Justice Mustill draws a number of contrasts in this passage. The mother is portrayed as concerned only about finance, while the professionals are seen as altruistic and thought to have gone beyond the call of duty in their commitment to the vital business of saving lives. The incident that might have harmed the boy concerned was regarded as a single lapse, uncharacteristic of their general excellence and dedication. That dedication was revered and the fact that litigation challenged it was seen as a reason for denying liability. There is an implicit acceptance that professionals are not to be equated with the health service that employs them. The latter would be fair game for litigation, but professionals make a personal contribution whose importance is captured in the evocative language of the navigation of 'perilous shoals' that are a matter of life and death.

    The law has built on this image of professionalism to construct a model of healthcare law that assumes and promotes the moral basis of medical practice (Montgomery 2006). This has been particularly explicitly articulated by Lord Donaldson, who has sought to explain that the law constructs a partnership between patient and professional whereby the moral integrity of both is maintained.

No one can *dictate* the treatment to be given to any child, neither court, parents nor doctors. ... The doctors can recommend treatment A in preference to treatment B. They can also refuse to adopt treatment C on the grounds that it is medically contra-indicated or for some other reason is a treatment which they could not conscientiously administer. The court or parents for their part can refuse to consent to treatment A or B or both, but cannot insist on treatment C. The inevitable and desirable result is that choice of treatment is in some measure a joint decision of the doctors and the court or parents. (Re J 1991:934)

In constructing this partnership, Donaldson is keen to recognise a moral as well as technical basis for the professional role – hence the reference to conscience. Thus, in one controversial area, he saw the existence of an internal medical ethic as justifying the creation of considerable discretion in doctors as to whether to accept the decisions of young women (under the age of 18) when their parents took a different view. This led him to permit the consent of either the woman or the parents to justify treatment. When it was suggested that this would allow abortion to be imposed upon a young woman who wanted to keep her child, he countered with the fact that he was confident that medical ethics would not permit it (Re W 1992:31). He thought that the alternative view would place doctors in the 'intolerable' position of being sued or prosecuted if they made an incorrect legal judgment as to who to go to for consent. He set out to establish a framework under which the 'doctor will be presented with a professional and ethical but not a legal problem' (Re R 1991:185).

This arms-length regulation of medicine has been described as an abdication of responsibility by the judiciary. José Miola argues that 'medical ethics has been allowed to take over from medical law' on the assumption 'that there are in existence rules and sanctions available to medical ethics to, first, judge the behaviour of the medical practitioner and, secondly, to be able to discipline him/her if necessary' (Miola 2004, pp. 262–263). He shows how such guidance is not always determinative. He sees this as a fault – 'what is left ... is a regulatory vacuum that can only be filled by the individual morality of the individual medical practitioner. If medical law and medical ethics are to serve any kind of purpose at all, this must be seen as clear evidence of their failure to discharge it.' However, it can also be seen as a deliberate strategy to integrate law and professional ethics into a single system based around a common purpose to which clinical freedom is directed (Montgomery 2006). We therefore need to consider how clinical freedom should be understood in the context of competing versions of professionalism.

Clinical freedom: a negative or positive right?

The problem can be illuminated by considering the concept of 'clinical freedom' in the light of a strand of philosophical debate about the nature of freedom and liberty. Isaiah Berlin drew attention to the difference between negative and positive conceptions of liberty (Berlin 1969). The negative concept of liberty stressed the importance of people being free from coercion by others – protecting individuals from having their actions restricted by the state. He compared this with the idea of positive liberty, the freedom to do things. Proponents of positive conceptions of liberty point out that negative liberty protects those who already have the means and ability to exercise their freedom, but does nothing to ensure that all citizens have at least a minimal opportunity to benefit from their liberties. Positive conceptions of liberty require the investment of state resources to guarantee freedom to act, not merely to police against intrusions by others.

Part of Berlin's argument was that political movements that were built around the concept of positive freedom too easily collapsed into a form of tyranny that imposed a particular version of the good life upon people, even on those who did not share that vision. However, in a context where the rationale for building a legal system around a concept of professionalism is built on the fact that the professions develop a normative value system that it is desirable to reinforce, then it becomes clear the negative conception of professional liberty is insufficient to deliver the benefits sought. The reason for protecting clinical freedom through the law is not to protect professionals from interference (a negative claim) but to ensure that these professional values can be acted upon (a positive claim). Thus, the proper claim to be made is not one that health professionals should be self-regulating and free from external control, but one that the law should ensure that they are free to act professionally on behalf of those they serve.

'Clinical freedom' should not therefore be seen as a slogan behind which medical power should be hidden (a negative conception of freedom *from* accountability) but as the foundation on which the service that health professionals give their patients is based (freedom *to* exercise clinical judgement). Assessment of the proper meaning and extent of clinical freedom should be made by reference to its contribution to that purpose. One way in which this positive conception of clinical freedom has become manifest is in the context of professional regulation. Doctors are generally not permitted to practise without a licence from their regulatory body. A model based on freedom from accountability would be characterized by a system which defined the boundaries of acceptable behaviour (punishing those who transgressed them by removing their licence to practise) but gave little consideration to what practitioners did within the scope of those boundaries. On this model, provided that doctors do not overstep those limits, their practice should remain largely immune to external challenge.

This was very much the picture in the UK prior to 1995. Until that date, the General Medical Council's guidance on professional conduct and discipline (known as the 'Blue Book') was primarily concerned with setting out the type of misbehaviour that might call into question a doctor's continuing registration. Since then the focus has changed, and a series of documents under the umbrella title of 'Duties of a Doctor' introduced a very different approach that set out the content of 'Good Medical Practice'. This marked a fundamental shift in the nature of professional regulation; *from* resistance against external scrutiny of clinical judgement on the basis of claims to professional autonomy, *to* explicitly asserting the principles on which the legitimacy of clinical freedom was based. The enforcement of compliance to these principles through professional disciplinary processes provides a justification for continuing the regulatory processes. It provides assurance to society that the clinical freedom that it provides for medical professionals will in fact deliver the type of professional service that it requires. This can be seen as a positive strategy for asserting professional independence, similar to that followed by nursing (Montgomery 1998), as well as a defensive reaction to scandals that have undermined confidence in self-regulation (Irvine *et al.* 2010).

A parallel development can be seen in the growth of evidence-based medicine and the associated expansion in the use of clinical guidelines. Here, the codification of expertise leads to a conception of clinical freedom based on the substance of what should be done, rather than deference to individuals who have received professional training. It shifts the nature of the claims made in the name of clinical freedom away from trust in the individual expertise of doctors towards the implementation of collective wisdom; less the assertion of occupational power than the deployment of scientific knowledge. Where such evidence exists and has been codified into guidelines, then claims to clinical freedom are generally judged against compliance with established best practice. Thus, in malpractice litigation, courts will regard departure from guidelines as providing preliminary evidence that proper professional practice has not been followed. This will not automatically indicate legal liability, but the doctor will need to show that their departure from the protocol was in fact the right thing to do in the circumstances (Montgomery 2003, pp. 183–184).

Clinical freedom in UK mental health legislation

These developments in the claims for clinical freedom can be seen with a slightly different emphasis in the context of mental health law. A number of pressures have led the law relating to psychiatry to develop separately from other areas of healthcare law. These include the earlier expression of scepticism against the evidence base for psychiatry than other areas of medicine, particularly the anti-psychiatry movement of the 1960s. There is also the greater likelihood for tension between the expressed wishes of patients and clinical assessments of their best interests in cases where capacity and autonomy may be impaired by mental illness. There is also a tension between public protection and individual interests, although this features more strongly in the minds of politicians than the evidence warrants. These factors are exacerbated in the context of the use of compulsion for personal and/or public protection. This raises significant human rights concerns, not least in the shadow of awareness of the abuse of psychiatry as a tool for social control in some totalitarian regimes. Claims to clinical freedom are therefore more complex in psychiatry than in other areas. The evidence base for clinical practice is regarded with greater suspicion than for other medical specialties; there is concern for the protection of individuals against coercion and the public against poorly understood (and often overestimated) risk.

Changes in mental health law over time generally reflect the prevailing understanding of the nature of psychiatry (Unsworth 1987), and the current framework of English mental health law (Mental Health Act 1983, as amended by the Mental Health Act 2007) can be used to illustrate how the contemporary understanding of the nature of professional power influences the way in which it is regulated. Some of its features show how, in this area of law, medical professionalism is unusually constrained by lay oversight. However, it can also be seen how these constraints shape rather than limit the exercise of clinical judgement. Where expertise is directed at balancing the key issues that society recognizes, then doctors are free to exercise it. The aim is to protect clinical freedom to act in the best interests of patients and society.

The Act structures the decisions to be taken by psychiatrists in two ways, in each case respecting clinical freedom by not dictating the outcome of the decision and accommodating the possibility that different views might be taken of the best way forward. The first mechanism for structuring clinical decisions is by specifying the questions to be asked. Thus, for detention for treatment under Section 3 of the Act, three questions must be addressed by the psychiatrist. The first is clinical: whether there is a diagnosis of mental disorder of a nature or degree making hospital treatment appropriate. Unless such a clinical diagnosis is made, then detention will not be lawful. The second concerns the balancing of risks. Clinicians need to ask whether hospital treatment is necessary in the interest either of the health or safety of the patient, or for the protection of other people. Even where this is the case, detention is only lawful if the treatment would not be provided unless the patient was detained. The third question is whether appropriate treatment is available for the patient. Only if this is the case can patients be detained (although short-term detention for assessment may be possible under other provisions of the statute).

The second mechanism for structuring professional power lies in process constraints. Many of the medical powers recognized under the Mental Health Act need to be deployed through collaborative and interdisciplinary procedures. Thus, admission for treatment requires a second medical opinion, making the exercise of clinical freedom a collaborative rather than individual activity. Further, compulsory admission must be initiated by either the patient's 'nearest relative' or an approved mental health professional (usually a social worker). Thus, process constraints minimize the risk that detention will be for reasons other than the purposes set out in the legislation by ensuring that psychiatrists cannot act alone. Similarly, decisions on certain types of treatment under Part IV of the Act require consultation with second opinion doctors, nursing staff and also professional carers who are not medically or nursing qualified. However, they do not remove from the psychiatrist the responsibility for determining what treatment to give. Further observations can be made about the relative positions of different health professions in this legislation (Montgomery 1992), but the key point for this discussion is that the law seeks to direct clinical freedom to the goal for which it is recognized, not merely to establish an area of non-regulation.

This approach to structuring clinical freedom is driven by a desire to specify conditions under which it will be exercised for the purposes for which it is conferred by society; freedom to exercise judgement rather than freedom from scrutiny. Doctors are not permitted to do whatever they like, but they are given the power to deploy their skills in achieving the balance of rights and risks that society has identified as needing their expertise. Thus, the clinical freedom that is protected is freedom to deliver, not freedom from control. This can also be seen in the use of a Code of Practice so that guidance on good practice can be established with a degree of legislative authority but without the rigidity entailed by statutory provisions. Developing such a Code of Practice, in consultation with the profession, enables the freedom conferred by the law to be directed towards its purpose and uses legal regulation to encourage ways of practising rather than to catch out malpractice (Alderson and Montgomery 1996).

The final interesting feature of the English mental health legislation lies in the subjection of clinical freedom to lay oversight in managers' hearings and mental health review tribunals, now known in England as the 'First Tier Tribunal (Mental Health)'. This is one of the starkest differences between English mental health law and the more general healthcare law. Under Section 23 of the Mental Health Act 1983 (as amended) and Chapter 31 of the Mental Health Act Code of Practice (2008 edition), a panel of lay people can discharge from hospital a patient whom the clinician believes should be detained. While there is guidance on the questions that managers should address, there is nothing to indicate how they should treat divergence between their lay view and the professional opinions of psychiatrists, and this remains controversial (Kennedy 2000, Montgomery 2003, pp. 340–341). It is easier to see how the tribunals indicate the emergence of a new professionalism, providing a context for clinical freedom rather than either deferring to professional opinion or overriding it. Tribunals are tasked with ensuring that prolonged detention is justified against the criteria set out in the Act, but they are multidisciplinary, with legal, medical and lay members. Thus, they recognize that the issues are not solely clinical but ensure clinical insight in decision-making.

The development of a new professionalism

The collaborative decision-making procedures that mental health legislation establishes are the key to a modern defence of professionalism, pointing to the way in which the compact between professionals and the state is changing. As Johnson (1972) noted, one of the less palatable peculiarities of professionalism lay in the way that professionals determined not only what options were available to the clients, but also defined their problems for them. This created a context for the compact between state and profession in which the client, for us the patient, played a minimal role. They become the object over which professional power is exercised rather than the main protagonist in the relationship. In this way, high respect for medical professionalism is linked with disempowerment of patients. Indeed, the very word 'patient' implies that they are the passive recipient of professional largesse, the object of the contract between the state and the profession rather than the contracting party. This is particularly the case in the context of socialized medicine, where patients do not have a contracting relationship with their doctors. Rather the doctor's contract is with the state to provide services, on the terms agreed between the profession and the state, to patients. This situation is changing in a number of respects, and a new formulation of the contract between professional and state that gives patients a more central place has emerged. This both alters the nature of professionalism and also makes it more defensible.

The structure of professional employment in the NHS

The notion of a contract between profession and state is often no more than a metaphor that is used to illuminate the nature of the relationship, supposedly reciprocal and based on mutual benefit. In the context of a system for socialized medicine such as the UK's NHS, this is much more than a metaphor. The majority of doctors hold real legal contracts with the state. This provides an opportunity to see what understanding of the rights and responsibilities of professionals is written into those agreements and how the interplay between professional power, clinical freedom and service requirements is manifest in the terms of the contracts.

The work of general medical practitioners (GPs) is defined largely by a contract, set out in regulations (NHS (General Medical Services Contracts) Regulations 2004, SI 2004/291 as amended) but negotiated between government and the trade union leaders of the profession in the British Medical Association. While, in cases of deadlock, changes in the terms of the GP contract are occasionally imposed, it remains a clear example of a compact between the state and a profession. The doctors concerned are known as 'independent contractors' because although they work for the NHS, they are not formally employed by it. Prior to the early 1990s, the contract did little to specify the work that GPs were expected to do. Indeed, its main clause indicated that GPs were expected to offer such services as GPs usually provided – a self-referring definition that protected the power of GPs to define their own work. Since that time, the contract has been used by governments to incentivize changes in behaviour that it desired, beginning with rewards for high immunization rates and now mediated through the very detailed payment system for achieving various 'points' within the 'quality and outcomes framework'. It still, however, recognizes a high degree of professional autonomy, and the core obligation under the contract is to provide services for the medical management of patients 'in the manner determined by the practice in discussion with the patient' (article 15(3) of the 2004 Regulations).

Professional work has therefore become more closely defined by its state patrons than the traditional independence of the Parsonian paradigm. Some have described the consequences of closer control of professional work as undermining the very concept of the profession – deprofessionalizing the relevant occupational groups, or from the perspective of Marxist theorists of professionalism, a process of 'proletarianisation' (Turner 1995). As the work that doctors do becomes directed by employers in the same way as other jobs, then the differential status of 'professional' is diminished. This issue can be seen very clearly in the development of the contract of NHS medical consultants.

Historically, the contractual status of NHS consultants showed very clearly their professional independence from the day-to-day control of NHS managers. Four aspects of their terms of employment can capture the salient points and provide an opportunity to reflect on the way in which the position is developing. First, the contractual parties have changed. For many years, the legal contract was between the consultant and the relevant NHS Regional Health Authority, not between the consultant and the manager of the service in which they worked. Thus, direct managerial control of a consultant's work was limited by the fact that they were not the contractual employer. The contract was with the general representative of the state, not the specific hospital. This has changed, and the contractors are now the individual consultant and the NHS Trust or health authority for which they work. The position developed again in 2003 when, under the current NHS consultant contract, a specific 'job planning' process was negotiated, so that a consultant's contract will now include an agreement on how their time should be spent in terms of 'programmed activities'. Job plans vary considerably in their precision and comprehensiveness, but the essential point for the tracking of professionalism is that the consultant's manager now has the ability, backed up by the legal contract of employment, to see whether the consultant is working in the way expected.

Second, the mechanisms for enforcing the consultant contract when things go wrong and the consultant is in conflict with their employer have in the past looked very different from the more common employment contract. Usually, employers have the contractual powers to discipline and if necessary dismiss their employees. However, in the case of NHS consultants, there was until the 2003 contract a legally recognized buffer against direct managerial control that reflects the different professional status granted to the consultants. Under the earlier terms and conditions, a consultant had an appeal to the Secretary of State in disciplinary issues (under paragraph 190 of the consultant terms and conditions contained in a health service circular (HC(90)9), see Mandal v Rotherham NHST 2000). This has now been replaced by local disciplinary procedures (Chan v Barts and the London NHS Trust 2007).

Third, access to consultant status is effectively controlled by the profession through a nationally prescribed appointment process, set out in the law and therefore not within local control (NHS (Appointment of Consultants) Regulations 1996, as amended in 2004). This process ensures professional dominance. The relevant Royal College has to approve the job description, enabling the profession to veto changes that might be desired by local managers. Membership of 'advisory appointment panels' was previously prescribed to include almost exclusively existing medical consultants, but this has now been reduced to a majority. Thus, entry to the exalted status of 'consultant' was essentially, and may still be, within the patronage of the profession itself rather than its paymasters. Once again, professional autonomy was inscribed in the law but has more recently become more aligned with managerial structures.

Fourth, there is an unusual (possibly unique) remuneration system by which NHS consultants receive 'top-up' payments for performance over and above the requirements of their contract. When the NHS was created, the medical profession fought strongly against it, and amongst the tools used by the government of the day to win them over was money. Nye Bevan famously said that he had won the consultants over by 'stuffing their mouths with gold', permitting them to retain their private practice rights and introducing a system of 'merit awards' for those consultants judged most worthy by their peers. Consultants consolidated a regular income from the state without loss of their professional freedom (Timmins 1995:115). The merit award system provided a subset of consultants with significant additional remuneration above the contractual salary and has developed, through renaming as 'Distinction Awards', into the current Clinical Excellence Award (CEA) Scheme, for whose governance the author has been responsible since 2005.

Our interest for the purpose of this piece is in the way in which the changing nature of professionalism can be traced in the recent developments in the awards system. It enables us to track some of the features of a current form of the contract between professionals and state that go some way to illustrating the nature of a new professionalism. Most important are the reforms to the process by which consultants are selected for recognition. Prior to the introduction of the current scheme, Merit and Distinction Awards were conferred through a rather secretive process whereby consultants already in possession of an award considered the merits of those without and selected those they found most worthy for advancement (Kendell 1994). Under the framework set out in 2003 for consultants working in England and Wales (Scotland and Northern Ireland have separate schemes), the process begins with an application from the consultant in question, rather than 'nomination' by a third party (DH 2003). This moved the awards scheme from one based on internal professional patronage to one based on open competition, and it also facilitated a number of developments in decision-making processes that reflect a changing structure for professional power.

Evaluation of 'clinical excellence' for the purpose of the scheme is no longer in the exclusive hands of consultants. The subcommittees of the Advisory Committee on Clinical Excellence Awards (ACCEA) are balanced to comprise half consultant members of the profession, one quarter employer representatives (who may include some medical directors) and one quarter lay people. The recommendations of these subcommittees who score the applications against a published set of criteria (ACCEA 2009c) are a very strong predictor of the awards finally made by the Secretary of State (ACCEA 2009a). There is recognition of the fact that consultants are more like traditional employees in the fact that eligibility for the scheme now requires consultants to have participated in job planning and appraisal, and their employer has to confirm this and give their own evaluation of the consultant's contribution as part of the application process. The criteria for judging excellence have gradually developed to reflect the requirements of national policy, incorporating the drive for improved quality by requiring evidence from applicants of their work in these dimensions (ACCEA 2009b) and, for the first time in the Guides published for the 2010 round of applications, including markers of excellence that have been drawn up in consultation with patients (ACCEA 2009a).

What is happening here is what is currently described in the NHS as a process of 'co-production'. The old merit award system was run by doctors for doctors, enabling them to commit public funds without either accountability or transparency. The new system aligns the financial incentives with the needs of the NHS, as defined by it leaders, but retains a system of peer review that enables award holders to regard the making of a clinical excellence award as an indication of esteem and not merely a bribe for accommodating managerial demands. The extension of the body of peers who are making the relevant judgements to include managers and lay people and the inclusion of such views in the development of criteria for excellence balance two fundamental dynamics that are essential to a version of professionalism that is needed in a modern health service. The profession continues to be able to develop its standards and values, removed from the immediate concerns of day-to-day management. This gives patients confidence that professionals can stand up for their interests against short-term political or financial expediency. The consultant contract alone risks this development because job plans are agreed and enforced locally without regard to their broader implications. Balanced with the CEA Scheme, there is proper scope for professional independence. The integration of the scheme with national policy developments and the involvement of lay people and managers in the evaluation process prevent the system becoming a bastion of professional privilege that insulates consultants from the need to demonstrate that freedom for them is the foundation for service for others. The exercise of clinical freedom in the interests of patients is rewarded.

Conclusions

This chapter has shown that the concept of 'professionalism' can be defined in a number of different ways, with both positive and negative resonances. Lawmakers have absorbed the virtues of a benign vision of the self-image of the profession into their thinking, but in doing so have sometimes reinforced an unattractive version of professionalism as a form of occupational power. As the realization of this transfiguration from virtue into vice has dawned, a cynicism about professionalism has led to an attack on self-regulation and an over-optimistic faith in the doctrinal resources of the law, especially the concept of rights, to redress the balance (Montgomery 1996, 2006). This development is also based on an impoverished understanding of the nature of professionalism.

What is required is the recognition of the power of the metaphor that professional status is built on a contract between the profession and the society it serves, which has very concrete forms in the case of UK medicine, to provide a mechanism to move forward. The vices of professionalism come to the fore when a profession is able to dictate the terms of the contract and prevent society ensuring that it gets what it bargained for. To counteract these vices with the promotion of consumerism risks as much as it gains. Consumerism is fundamentally amoral. It regards the customer as king irrespective of the acceptability of their motivation and reduces the service provider to an unreflective responder to consumer desires without recognition of the personal integrity of the individuals working in the service (Montgomery 1996). This is a model that poorly reflects the motivations of professionals, the nature of the social contract upon which the National Health Service rests (currently enshrined in the NHS Constitution, with its recognition of roles and responsibilities of both patients and staff), or the expectations of patients of high-quality care.

If traditional professionalism enables the profession to dictate the terms of the contract between state and profession, the same problem emerges if the pendulum swings so far as to enable consumers to dictate the terms without regard to the integrity of the profession. Instead, we need a contract that offers both professionals and patients an accommodation that reflects mutual benefits. The freedoms that the law provides professionals must not be based on freedom *from* managerial interference, but instead set out the conditions that confer the freedom *to* provide the services that patients, professionals and policy-makers have together defined as the proper purpose of (in our case) medicine.

The Royal College of Physicians working party report argued that the values it had identified as the essence of modern professionalism – integrity, compassion, altruism, continuous improvement, excellence and working in partnership with members of the wider healthcare team – formed 'the basis for a moral contract between the medical profession and society. Each party has a duty to work to strengthen the system of healthcare on which our collective human dignity depends.' (Royal College of Physicians 2005a:45). This chapter has examined how such a social contract has been inscribed into English law and how it might be revised to meet the needs of a modern professionalism that benefits us all.

References

Advisory Committee on Clinical Excellence Awards (2009a). *Annual Report 2009 Round.* London: ACCEA.

Advisory Committee on Clinical Excellence Awards (2009b). *Guide for Applicants.* London: ACCEA.

Advisory Committee on Clinical Excellence Awards (2009c). *Guide for Assessors.* London: ACCEA.

Alderson P, Montgomery J (1996). *Heath Care Choices: Making Decisions with Children.* London: Institute for Public Policy Research.

Berlin I (1969). Two concepts of liberty. In *Four Essays on Liberty.* Oxford: Oxford University Press.

Bolam v W Friern HMC [1957]. 2 All England Reports 118.

Bolitho v City & Hackney HA [1997]. 4 All England Reports 771.

Chan v Barts and the London NHS Trust [2007]. England & Wales High Court 2914.

De Freitas v O'Brien [1995]. 6 Medical Law Reports 108.

Department of Health (2003). *The New NHS Consultant Reward Scheme: Clinical Excellence Awards.* London: DH.

Hucks v Cole (1960) [1994]. 4 Medical Law Reports 393.

Irvine D, Johnson N, Thistlethwaite J, Lewando Hundt G (2010). Professionalism: the UK perspective. In D Bhugra, A Malik (eds.) *Professionalism in Mental Healthcare: Experts, Expertise and Expectations.* New York: Cambridge University Press, pp. 48–61.

Kendell R (1994). *Report of the Working Party on the Review of the Consultants Distinction Awards Scheme.* Leeds: NHS Executive, issued with EL(94)99.

Kennedy H (2000). Managers' hearings: dialectic and maternalism. *Psychiatric Bulletin* 24, 361–362.

Johnson T (1972). *Professions and Power.* Basingstoke: Macmillan.

Mahon v Osborne [1939]. 1 All England Reports 535.

Mandal v Rotherham NHST [2000]. 58 Butterworths Medico-Legal Reports 112.

Maynard v West Midlands RHA [1985]. 1 All England Reports 635.

Miola J (2004). Medical law and medical ethics – complementary or corrosive? *Medical Law International* 6, 251–274.

Montgomery J (1989). Medicine, accountability and professionalism. *Journal of Law and Society* 16, 319–339.

Montgomery J (1992). Doctors handmaidens: the legal contribution. In S McVeigh, S Wheeler (eds.) *Law, Health and Medical Regulation.* Aldershot: Dartmouth.

Montgomery J (1996). Patients first: the role of rights. In K Fulford, S Errser, A Hope (eds.) *Essential Practice in Patient-Centred Care.* Oxford: Blackwell Science, 142–152.

Montgomery J (1998). Professional regulation: a gendered phenomenon? In S Sheldon, M Thomson (eds.) *Feminist Perspectives in Health Care Law.* London: Cavendish, 33–51.

Montgomery J (2000). Time for a paradigm shift? Medical law in transition. *Current Legal Problems* 53, 363–408.

Montgomery J (2003). *Health Care Law.* Oxford: Oxford University Press.

Montgomery J (2006). Law and the demoralisation of medicine. *Legal Studies* 26, 185–210.

Parsons T (1939). The professions and the social structure. *Social Forces* 17, 457.

Re J [1991]. 3 All England Reports 930.

Re R [1991]. 4 All England Reports 177.

Re W (1992). 9 Butterworths Medico-Legal Reports 22.

Royal College of Physicians (2005a). *Doctors in Society: Medical Professionalism in a Changing World.* Report of a Working Party of the Royal College of Physicians of London. London: RCP.

Royal College of Physicians (2005b). *Doctors in Society: Medical Professionalism in a Changing World.* Technical Supplement to a Report of a Working Party of the Royal College of Physicians of London. London: RCP.

Scarman L (1987). Law and medical practice. In P Byrne (ed.) *Medicine in Contemporary Society*. London: King Edwards Fund for London, 131–139.

Sidaway v Bethlem RHG [1985]. 1 All England Reports 643.

Timmins N (1995). *The Five Giants: A Biography of the Welfare State*. London: HarperCollins.

Turner B (1995). *Medical Power and Social Knowledge*. London: Sage Publications.

Unsworth C (1987). *The Politics of Mental Health Legislation*. Oxford: Oxford University Press.

Wilsher v Essex AHA [1986]. 3 All England Reports 801.

Woolf H (2001). Are the courts excessively deferential to the medical profession? *Medical Law Review* **9**, 1.

Professionalism
The US perspective

Sidney Weissman and Kenneth Busch

Editors' introduction

The American healthcare system has several types of providers, leading to a plethora of mini-systems, all of which have different pitfalls as well as advantages. Working within each of these systems brings with it specific issues of definition, training and delivery of services. In spite of a large proportion of the gross domestic product (GDP) being devoted to healthcare delivery, approximately one sixth of the population is uninsured and has access only to emergency treatments.

In this chapter, Weissman and Busch provide a historical account of the development of the healthcare system in the United States and the role of various reports and organizations in defining medical professionalism. Changes in organized medicine in response to the demands of society and changing public expectations have led us to revisit the components of medical professionalism. Training in medical schools and at trainee level has been redesigned to make psychiatrists aware of issues related to medical professionalism. The number of doctors belonging to various professional organizations is poor at national level, but not necessarily at state or local levels. This indicates that local issues matter more to physicians. In addition, access to psychological treatment has become less readily available, largely because of resource constraints. The interaction between the society and the individual doctor is also influenced by events such as war and system changes related to both the healthcare payment system and the federal healthcare systems. Society takes on the responsibility of looking after its sick and vulnerable members, and doctors in turn are responsible for monitoring the standards of medical education and healthcare delivery. Medical professionalism must respond to these challenges.

Introduction

In recent years the concept of professionalism has undergone a rapid extension. It once was restricted to areas such as medicine or law – areas where a unique set of abilities was critical to becoming a member of the profession, and the profession had a unique standing in society and unique responsibilities to society. Upon becoming a member of a profession, each individual assumed a number of explicit responsibilities to both their profession and the individuals upon or for whom they applied their specific skills. Members of these professions in turn were given special status by society. The concept of professionalism also applies to the conduct of the profession and refers to how the profession governs itself. Generally the

Professionalism in Mental Healthcare: Experts, Expertise and Expectations, ed. Dinesh Bhugra and Amit Malik. Published by Cambridge University Press. © Cambridge University Press 2011.

members of a profession decide on how the profession should be governed. The profession decides on who can become members and sets the standards for maintenance of membership. It further establishes the educational standards as to the knowledge and skill essential to practise the profession. For a profession to survive in a society, it requires the existence of a mutually agreed association between the society and the profession. We will focus on the broad aspect of medical professionalism rather than focus more narrowly on professionalism in psychiatry. The professional behaviour of psychiatrists as a branch of medicine is predominantly shaped by its parent profession. In this chapter we will review how medical professionalism has evolved to its present state in the United States and make recommendations for its ongoing survival.

To accomplish this task we will utilize the classic definition of the concept of 'professional' as it relates to an individual's action as well as to the structure and governance of the profession and the profession's relationship to society (see also Chapter 1). Other uses of the term, although now widely applied, do not address the unique responsibilities required by members of a profession held by the classic use of the term 'profession'. For example, the professional athlete is seen as having more skill than the amateur and earns his living by practising his sport. Parts of the classic definition may apply to the professional athlete, but clearly not all.

The relationship of the medical profession with society

In the United States many professions have a strong connection to society. Neither courts nor legislative bodies claim to have the expertise to address professional matters. This principle of professional autonomy is generally followed, with one major exception. That is when one profession perceives that its right to practise or its scope of practice is or was interfered with or restricted by another. In these cases the courts have become involved to adjudicate these disputes. Examples of judicial interference can be seen in courts dealing with the scope of practice of osteopathic physicians and chiropractors. Today osteopathic physicians have the same rights and responsibilities as allopathic physicians, primarily because of the outcome of judicial action. State legislative bodies may and do at times also initiate actions which impact on the functioning and scope of the practice of professions. For example, in all 50 US states, legislative action expanded the scope of practice of optometrists to legally allow them to use diagnostic medications. At one time only physicians could prescribe or use these medications. In some states additional legislation was passed which allows optometrists to prescribe therapeutic medications.

Occasionally a profession works with society through complex governmental activities to address the unique areas of special concern related to the profession's expertise. However, the profession is at its strongest when because of its concerns it acts proactively to identify and address issues affecting it and society at large. An example of a professional organization initiating action with great impact on the society at large can be seen in the activities of the American Medical Association (AMA), the national medical membership organization founded in 1847. In 1908, when only 25% of American physicians belonged to it (American Medical Association Archives 2009), the AMA commissioned a report without general public concern or input to assess the educational structure and ownership of all American and Canadian medical schools (Flexner 1910). The AMA felt that, with the enhanced knowledge needed by physicians to effectively care for patients, major changes were needed in medical education to ensure physician competence to address the healthcare needs of Americans. It requested the Carnegie Foundation for the Advancement of Teaching to undertake a study of American medical education by reviewing the functioning of all American and Canadian medical schools. This report, issued in 1910, was named after its author, Abraham Flexner (Flexner 1910). It was used to support arguments for major changes in American medical education and subsequently American healthcare.

The AMA through its national and state associations after the publication of the Flexner Report worked with state legislatures to act to further enhance the quality of American medicine by developing standards for licensure of physicians. While the profession through the AMA used its authority to establish the standards of education for membership and subsequent entry into medical practice, each individual state established its own mechanisms of licensure. In 1921 a group of states founded the Federation of State Licensing Boards to attempt to bring about common standards between the states. This critical step would not have taken place without the AMA's prior independent action. By the 1930s, because of the Flexner Report, the last proprietary medical schools in the United States were closed.

Another example of the relationship between society and the profession of medicine is their collusion in the nineteenth and part of the twentieth century in the treatment of individuals with mental illness. At a time when there were limited therapeutic options for the treatment of the mentally ill, each state established and funded hospital systems which collectively housed thousands of patients suffering from mental illness. Even though most were inadequately funded, state-run mental health systems at the end of the nineteenth century were large state government enterprises that consumed vast portions of state budgets. Unfortunately, state mental hospitals were the major employer in some communities, leading to the politicization of mental healthcare in those states. The standards for care in these state hospitals were frequently controlled through political appointments outside of the power or influence of organized medicine.

At the same time organized medicine appeared to look the other way. The psychiatric profession was not strong enough on its own to bring about reform. In any event many states allowed unlicensed physicians to care for the mentally ill in these hospitals. Serious patient abuse still occurs in some state-run systems today. In 2009 the Atlanta Journal and Constitution published a series of articles describing abuse of mentally ill patients in Georgia state-run mental hospitals (A. Miller, personal communication, 2009; Atlanta Journal and Constitution 2009). Nowadays, although stigma is still attached to mental illness, there is a clearer acceptance of responsibility to meet the needs of the mentally ill in American society.

In 2008 the United States Congress passed and the president signed a law requiring health insurance plan parity or equality between the funding of care provided for physical disorders and coverage provided for mental disorders. This reform was accomplished by political activism generated by the American Psychiatric Association (APA), the AMA and patient advocacy groups. This was an excellent instance of physician and patient groups working together to meet societal needs.

The first definition of a medical professional

In medicine one of the first representations of the profession and its unique values is in the writings of Hippocrates and in the Hippocratic Oath (Ludwig 1943). The oath presents the unique demands and expectations that are placed on the healer. Although elements of the oath relate to the time it was originally written, the cardinal relationship between healer and patient and the responsibilities of the healer are clearly stated. The healer must do no harm to their patients (non-maleficence), provide good care for their patient (beneficence), respect their patient's autonomy and have responsibilities to society. Further the responsibilities of the healer to his profession are also stated by Hippocrates. 'To hold him who has taught me this are as equal to my parents and to live my life in partnership with him, and if he is in need of money to give him a share to mine …' (Ludwig 1943). While far removed from today's physician and his relationship to his teachers, the words demonstrate a traditional relationship between the physician and their responsibilities to the profession. Without teachers we would not have a profession. Today the oath has been rewritten. A modern version of the oath written by Louis Lasagna in 1964 is used by graduates of a number of medical schools (Lasagna 1964) and explicitly addresses issues related to the practice of modern medicine and the role of the medical profession in society, with a clearer sense of the role of science.

Change in organized medicine and its impact on professionalism

The AMA and the Flexner Report 1910

In the United States medicine is perceived as a powerful scientific and economic profession, but for over the first 100 years of the nation's history many physicians were either ill-trained or, frankly, charlatans. In 1904 the AMA created its Council on Medical Education (CME). The council was founded with the objective of restructuring American medical education and improving medical practice and the health of the nation. At its first annual meeting, the council adopted two principles, to establish minimal standards for acceptance into medical schools and to outline medical school curricula. In 1908, the CME asked the Carnegie Foundation to survey American medical schools to develop data which would enable it to reform medical education. The Carnegie Foundation selected Abraham Flexner to conduct the survey.

Flexner visited the 155 medical schools in the United States and Canada. Most were proprietary and existed to make profits for their owners. Prior to the Flexner Report, anyone could pay a fee and become or at least be called a doctor. The Flexner Report, building on the AMA CME standards, established the framework in the United States for the structure of medical school education (Flexner 1910). To a great extent, the model it proposed 100 years ago is still the template of American medical school education. Medical schools were not to be for-profit undertakings but part of universities. Medical school curricula would be based on 2 years of basic science and 2 years in teaching hospitals. In 1914, building on its work with medical schools, the AMA CME developed the first standards for a 1-year post-medical school training experience referred to as an internship.

By 1936 there were only 65 medical schools in the United States and Canada. When Flexner produced his report in 1910, only 16 of 155 schools or 10% required applicants to have 2 or more years of college. By 1920 the number was 92% (American Medical Association Archives 2009). The actions of the AMA in the early years of the last century showed it to be at the peak of its authority as the professional association representing the needs of medicine, its practitioners and society at large rather than protecting the status quo for a privileged few. By its actions, the AMA upheld the values of Hippocrates of serving society as well as learning to do no harm to one's patients by enhancing the quality of medical education.

American medicine after the Flexner Report: the rise of specialization and the profession's response

As medicine became more sophisticated, post-medical school internship training expanded to include postgraduate training or residency training. This included a number of years of primarily hospital-based training in a specific medical discipline. Residency training further evolved into still more focused post-residency training called fellowship training. With the development of specialized training came a need to set standards for performance and ability in the evolving medical specialties. In the absence of a Flexner-type report on graduate medical education, medical specialties developed 'boards' or certifying bodies to determine the abilities of specialists in their specific area. The first specialty board in the United States was the American Board of Ophthalmology incorporated in 1917, followed by the American Board of Otolaryngology incorporated in 1924. In 1933 the American Board of Medical Specialties (ABMS) was incorporated to serve as the umbrella organization for the development of appropriate universal standards for the initial certification of physicians upon completion of specialty and for future boards (American Board of Medical Specialties Annual Report 2000). Today the ABMS also sets standards for how physicians who are certified may demonstrate their sustained competence by maintaining certification. For many years the ABMS had limited power, essentially serving as an administrative and record-keeping body. Today, with a focus on developing competencies in each field throughout a practitioner's clinical lifetime, the ABMS has attained enhanced power and authority and requires individual specialty boards to follow explicit requirements for its diplomates to retain certification.

In the United States it is not essential to obtain board certification in one's area of specialization in order to practise after completing a residency. In fact, board certification is not required in any state to obtain a licence to practise medicine. Some hospitals, however, will require physicians to obtain board certification in their requisite specialty in order to become members of their medical attending staff.

While the AMA still plays a part in the governance of the individual specialty boards and the ABMS, its role has declined with the passage of time. The AMA is only one of a number of organizations that nominate or appoint members to the ABMS or individual specialty boards. Those members nominated or appointed by the AMA do not have enough votes for the AMA to have a veto power over the actions of the ABMS or the individual specialty boards. In the United States this is but one example of how the AMA's central and once-dominant role in the internal professional regulation of medicine has declined.

The initial focus on credentialing graduates of specialty residency training programmes through specialty boards and the ABMS highlighted a need to monitor and accredit residency training programmes. This led to the development of a group to accredit residency training programmes, initially under the aegis of the AMA. This group started as the Liaison Committee for Graduate Medical Education in 1972, and in 1981 it became the Accreditation Council for Graduate Medical Education (ACGME) (Accreditation Council for Graduate Medical Education 2009). Over time the AMA lost a portion of its critical input as the Council evolved and became free-standing rather than being a component of the AMA.

Another decline in AMA authority occurred in 1943 when, in conjunction with the Association of American Medical Colleges (AAMC), it established the Liaison Committee for Medical Education (LCME) (Liaison Committee on Medical Education 2009). Here the AMA was joined by the AAMC in sustaining medical educational standards for medical schools, a role completely controlled by the AMA at one time.

The ABMS, the ACGME and the LCME – all with critical but varied areas of regulatory authority over elements of American medicine – were created outside of state or federal government control. They are completely sustained and regulated by a variety of medical associations. Key functions of each organization were once essentially totally controlled or performed by the AMA, but today the AMA plays a more limited role in these areas. The actions of these groups, committees or councils that deal with the broad areas of medical education impact on all states. For example, the LCME has the authority to accredit medical schools in all states, and the ACGME accredits residency training programmes in all states.

State medical societies or associations

Each state has its own medical society or medical association separate from the AMA. These societies are generally not mini-AMAs but are frequently more narrowly focused on medical guild-type issues in their respective state and are affiliated with the AMA. They will actively lobby state legislatures to support their views. They will work to limit or block the expansion of practice of non-MDs into areas which are or were traditionally performed by MDs. To accomplish this and other goals, lobbyists are hired to present their position to legislators. Society members will also directly lobby or meet with state legislators on their own either in their districts or the state capital to oppose legislation which they feel will interfere with the practice of medicine or to support legislation that will enhance the practice of medicine.

Besides political action in legislative areas, state societies also address areas of licensure or professional regulation in each state. They will work with state regulatory bodies to develop disciplinary boards to review the functioning of physicians on issues related to fitness to practice. Another example of their work is developing administrative and clinical practice policies related to state-run health programmes for individuals with limited financial resources.

Practitioners and medical societies

At the time the Flexner Report was written in 1910, 25% of all US physicians were members of the AMA (American Medical Association Archives 2009). Considering that large numbers of these physicians were graduates of marginal schools, AMA membership would have bestowed on them a sense of being part of the medical profession. AMA membership peaked in 1960 at 74.5% (American Medical Association Archives 2009). Today AMA membership is between 30 and 35%. Membership in state medial societies varies. It is highest in rural states. In New Mexico, a predominantly rural state, it is 85% (G. R. Marshall, personal communication, 2010), while in Illinois, an industrial state, it is 32% (C. Caine, personal communication, 2009).

Unlike in 1910, when medical society membership may have provided a core identity with the profession of medicine, membership today may be more related to relationships among peers. In urban areas a major medical peer group for practitioners is their hospital staff, who provide an important model for professional behaviour. In rural areas with small hospital staffs, doctors are more likely to feel isolated and look to the state medical society to provide peer relationships and models of professional behaviour. It is also the case that in rural areas doctors are more likely to be in primary care and not have specialty society interactions.

The lack of many physicians' affiliation with the AMA reduces its political authority and its impact on practice behaviour. This is especially significant because it limits the AMA's authority as a national stakeholder at a crucial time when the United States is examining healthcare reform in 2009. Further, it reduces the authority of the AMA's Council on Ethical and Judicial Affairs (CEJA), which still writes and sets the ethical standards for all American physicians and can potentially have a significant impact on professional behaviour.

Specialization and specialty societies

In addition to the AMA as the national presence of medicine as a profession, a number of national medical specialty organizations serve their members independently of the AMA. In some specialties, practitioners are likely to be members of their own specialty professional association and not the AMA. Psychiatry is a prime example. About two thirds of all psychiatrists are members of the American Psychiatric Association (APA), but significantly less than half are members of the AMA (AMA Physician Census 2007, APA 2009). Specialty associations include groups such as the American College of Physicians, the American College of Surgeons, the American Academy of Family Physicians, the American Academy of Pediatrics and the APA.

These organizations are national membership associations composed of physicians who completed residency training in their specific specialty. Board certification in the specific specialty to demonstrate competence is not usually required for association membership. Some of these associations have local or state affiliates which are either separate legal entities or direct branches of the national organizations.

These organizations through their national leadership nominate or appoint members to the respective boards that certify the competence of members of their specialty. They also appoint members to the section of the ACGME which develops standards for residency training in their specialty. They have critical roles in developing policies and standards for training and standards for competence in each specialty. Today these groups have an additional mission. Organized medicine has taken on the role of ensuring that Board Certified Practitioners demonstrate their competence periodically throughout their practice life under pressure from society to ensure the ongoing competence of practising physicians. The various boards, under the direction and guidance of the ABMS, are developing mechanisms to accomplish this. Being a modern-day medical professional will mean not only obtaining competence in the specific specialty by completing residency training but also demonstrating and maintaining competence throughout the tenure of one's practice.

Subspecialization

In 2000 the ABMS recognized 89 different subspecialties (American Board of Medical Specialties Annual Report 2000). A few of these specialties, such as sports medicine, could be practised by members of separate specialties. Since then a number of others have been added. Individuals who have obtained training in a subspecialty frequently form or join their own subspecialty organizations. When this occurs they frequently do not sustain membership in a specialty organization or a local or national medical society. Their focus in a subspecialty may be narrowed to its area of practice. Broader issues of their specialty or in the total quality of healthcare of the society may not be the subspecialist's focus or interest. In some subspecialties this can be partially understood, as the practitioner must sustain and focus attention to maintain the skill set to perform complex procedures. When society perceives the focus as assuring a high income level rather than learning and sustaining the ability to retain competence to perform procedures, this may not be seen as an advancement of professional responsibility. In turn these practitioners may lose interest in the broader issues of professionalism. They may function or at least be perceived as less like members of the medical profession with a responsibility for the healthcare of society and more like members of a guild protecting their practice and incomes from encroachment by other practitioners (Gawande 2009).

Special issues in psychiatry

Prior to the Second World War, with the exception of a handful of psychiatrists, most American psychiatrists practised in state-run mental hospitals with limited resources. Psychiatry in those settings focused on the treatment of psychosis and existed on the fringe of American medicine. A large number of psychoanalysts who fled Europe prior to or during the War established new lives in the United States. The entry of these practitioners coupled with the existence of the psychological horrors of the War placed a new emphasis on psychiatry. At the time, psychiatry became an important part of medicine. In many centres, psychoanalysis became the foundation of a new psychiatry. Within this background the primary treatment for patients became talking therapy. Talking therapies place special constraints on the psychiatrist which differ from the rest of medicine. Self-knowledge is seen as critical to be a psychiatrist, and many psychiatrists in this period felt it was essential to undergo a personal psychoanalysis or psychotherapy. Psychoanalysis was in many ways the dominant force in American psychiatry from the 1940s until the 1970s.

The 1960s saw the development of biological psychiatry with the introduction of new medications and of community-based treatment programmes. In the 1960s one of the most visible subspecialties of American psychiatry was the community psychiatrist. A split developed between community psychiatrists, who felt that they addressed psychiatry's responsibility to individuals with serious mental illness in community treatment programmes, while other psychiatrists in private practice treated individuals with less serious disorders. Differences in respective views of professional responsibility continue to exist today between both of these groups. An additional schism evolved between psychiatrists who focused on talking therapies and those on the use of medications.

Today, with the further development of numerous medications for treating mental illness, the focus on talking therapy has declined. Nowadays a major professional concern that most psychiatrists emphasize is privacy and confidentiality. With the development of the electronic medical record, the security of medical records has become a paramount concern. A unique professional concern for psychiatry is the process where a psychiatrist prescribes medication for a patient and either a social worker or psychologist provides the talking therapy. The professional responsibility for each practitioner is not always clear. For this reason and others, many psychiatrists do not adopt such an approach to treatment delivery where professional responsibilities are not always clear. These reasons also impact on the popularity of psychiatry as a specialty, and today only 4% of American medical students enter psychiatry (National Resident Matching Program 2009).

The impact of the shifting role of federal government and changing societal concerns on medical professionalism

The practice of medicine represents the outcome of the interaction between the profession of medicine and the values of the society. In the modern world the values of the society may evolve quite rapidly. In the United States it is the actions of the federal government which most clearly represent the values of the society. Individual practitioners and organized medicine must both respond to changes in society's values. In this section, broad changes in the policies of the American government which have impacted on healthcare in the past 100 years will be examined.

Overview

For the most part during this period, civilian healthcare was not a major concern of the federal government. The peak period for federal involvement in civilian healthcare issues occurred in the 1960s. In 1965 federal legislation created the Medicare and Medicaid programmes. Medicare provides insurance benefits for the elderly covered by Social Security and for disabled individuals. It is managed by a federal agency. The Medicaid programme provides the equivalent of health insurance for the poor or for chronically ill individuals who cannot work. These programmes were a major change in American healthcare and directly involved the federal government in healthcare programmes for ordinary civilians. Both the elderly and the poor now had a means of paying for healthcare from insurance. Previously, insurance existed only for those employed and their families. Significantly, the AMA opposed the passage of Medicare. Some feel this action fed a view that physicians were not concerned about the wellbeing of the public but were more concerned about their own financial interests. This in turn may have contributed to a lower opinion of doctors and a decline in authority and respect in the view of the public of the AMA.

For the past 20 years American medicine has seen attempts to increase efficiency and reduce cost. In 2008 the United States spent 16.2% of its GDP on healthcare (Centers for Medicare and Medicaid Services 2009). An additional concern has focused on the quality of healthcare.

This societal focus on healthcare brings about a problem for medicine in its relationship to society. Because professions exist in either a stated or unstated relationship with society, the profession and society must have shared values in order for this relationship to prosper. A tension arose between organized medicine and society when the former did not initially support Medicare and Medicaid, both of which received overwhelming societal support. The AMA, with the overwhelming authority of the government arrayed against it, eventually supported Medicare and now works in a number of ways to facilitate its effective functioning. On a state level, state medical societies in turn work to make Medicaid work – but the damage to medicine's reputation and prestige was done. Organized medicine was seen by some as not working for the public good. The capacity of organized medicine to work for the public good is what allows government to give organized medicine and the individual practitioner autonomy and authority to act.

Areas of interaction between society and medicine

War and physician shortage

At varying times special societal needs have intruded on American medicine, placing pressure on it to alter its self-determined standards. During the Second World War under federal government urging, medical school curricula in the United States were shortened to provide more physicians for the war effort in a short space of time. Immediately after the end of the War and without external pressure, medical school curricula reverted to pre-War standards. Later, after the War and fearing a major shortage, society called for a rapid increase in the production of physicians. Borrowing on the experience of the Second World War in order to quickly increase the supply of physicians, some American medical schools redesigned curricula so that medical students could graduate in 3 not 4 years. This was a short-lived experiment. The few schools that implemented the curricular changes did so without government interference or support and soon reverted back to 4-year curricula.

Healthcare payment systems

Payment systems for healthcare in the United States from early in the twentieth century to the 1930s led to the consolidation of essentially two kinds of general medical hospitals. Private non-profit hospitals frequently affiliated with religious organizations or medical schools and county or municipal hospitals. Individuals with some ability to pay were cared for at private hospitals, and the remaining citizens for the most part were treated in public hospitals, which were frequently the largest hospitals in the city.

In order to ensure funding for the private hospitals in the 1930s during the midst of the Depression, the hospital association developed an insurance system for individuals, which they named Blue Cross. Blue Cross was developed not with a primary intent of helping ill individuals or their families to pay for medical care in the hospital but to provide an assured revenue stream for the private hospitals. Physician payments were not included in the initial Blue Cross plan. Payments were paid to hospitals only for hospital care. Later a second system called Blue Shield was developed to provide payment for physicians' services provided in hospitals. Eventually these were expanded to also pay for physician services provided in the doctor's office. Today a variety of plans exist, marketed by an array of private insurance companies for payments to hospitals, physicians and laboratories.

At the conclusion of the Second World War when wage and price controls were in effect in the United States, unions and employers colluded to provide increases in employee benefits greater than those allowed by the then in existence wage control board. They accomplished this by fostering federal legislation that exempted employer payments for healthcare insurance to employees from taxable income. This led to the institutionalization of the current American system, where healthcare benefits for many are tied to employment. Organized medicine was not involved in these actions. In 1948 President Harry Truman proposed national government action on healthcare, which was promptly called socialized medicine by the AMA and politically conservative groups. At that time government action on developing universal healthcare was dropped. No major changes in the healthcare system for civilians occurred for many years after President Truman's initial efforts.

In 1965, with pressure from an aging population struggling to pay for healthcare, the United States Congress passed and President Lyndon Johnson signed a bill establishing Medicare. This legislation provides health coverage for citizens who participate in the Federal Social Security System and who are either over 65 years of age or suffer from a chronic illness. Besides providing health insurance coverage for the elderly, the Medicare programme did much more. It allowed the government, with the eventual co-operation of the AMA, to effectively set prices for all medical procedures used by patients with Medicare. These fees are generally significantly lower than usual private fees for service and the fees paid by many insurance companies. By these actions the federal government directly impacts on the practice of medicine provided to its citizens. The impact of Medicare on the healthcare system demonstrates society's power impacting upon a profession and how society can determine the economic success of the profession. As the country's largest healthcare payer, the US government now has a direct stake in the medical profession.

One example of its role which is not well known or understood is that the federal government plays a direct part in funding hospital-based residency programmes through the Medicare system. Direct payments are made to hospitals on a specific formula which is fixed by law and is independent of each year's federal budget process. By controlling through funding the number of residency positions, the government can exercise power in determining how many residency positions ought to exist. While the American government funds much of graduate medical education, it has shown little interest so far in interfering with curricula or directing medical education at any level or in determining the number of residents in a given specialty.

At the same time, the federal government also passed the Medicaid legislation. This programme is administered locally by each state and is funded equally by the state and federal government. The Medicaid programme was designed to give the poor and the chronically ill the equivalent of health insurance, which would pay for hospital and physician expenses and medication. Hospitals and physicians would agree to see a number of Medicaid patients at reduced fees. As long as the hospitals saw these patients in underused facilities, they could in fact make profits by providing patient care – but when the hospitals needed to add staff and facilities to care for these patients, they frequently lost money because of low compensation rates. Hospitals predominantly paid by Medicaid lose money, while other hospitals with a different payer mix may be quite profitable. While the Medicaid programme granted the poor access to hospitals other than the county or municipal hospitals that had previously been their major source of hospital care, it created a new set of underfunded hospitals. In light of this action, America has witnessed a growth of private hospitals and either a decline in the size of municipal hospitals or their complete closure. Today in most major American cities, university teaching hospitals are the largest and most prominent hospitals in the city.

The underfunding of Medicaid, with poor compensation rates for delivering services to poor patients, creates unique issues for physicians. Some will not treat these patients. Others give them less thorough treatment. In medical school hospitals, the care of patients on Medicaid is frequently given by residents and students and not the faculty. Thus, physicians indirectly contribute to the maintenance of a two-tier healthcare system based on the ability to pay.

In 1993 President Bill Clinton attempted to reform the American healthcare system. His proposals were met with opposition from organized medicine, the insurance industry and the pharmaceutical industry. Whilst his attempts failed, in 2009 another attempt was undertaken, this time with the support of organized medicine (the AMA) and the pharmaceutical industry. Compromise legislation was passed by the United States Congress in March 2010 and was signed into law by the president. This legislation became the first step in reforming the American healthcare system. It further established the principle that healthcare is a right for all Americans.

Federal healthcare systems

The federal government manages and owns three separate healthcare systems which provide direct patient care. The first is the military system, which provides care to active duty military personnel and their dependants and retirees and their dependants. Retirees are individuals who served 20 or more years on active duty in the United States Armed Forces. These services are provided in hospitals generally associated with military facilities around the world. Patients receiving treatment in these facilities do not make any payment for their care.

The government also runs a healthcare system for Native Americans. Again beneficiaries of this system do not pay for their care. This is the smallest of the three systems.

The largest government healthcare system is for military veterans. It provides ongoing treatment for veterans for injuries or illness acquired in military service. These disorders are referred to as service connected. It also provides general medical care to former soldiers who meet certain minimum income requirements and cannot afford private care.

The government-run Veterans' Affairs Hospitals serve thousands of people and act as a benchmark for models of care provided in the private sector. These hospitals also provide employment for thousands of healthcare workers. Frequently the loyalty of these physicians and their view of the medical profession and professionalism come from the Department of Veterans' Affairs and its value system, not the rest of medicine. Besides providing care, these hospitals also serve as major sites for the education of medical students and residents. The funding of residents in these hospitals is met by the Department of Veterans' Affairs and not by Medicare.

Issues in the cost of healthcare

In the past two decades medical decision-makers have focused on the cost of healthcare. The United States spends a greater percentage of its GDP on healthcare than any other industrialized nation (17% in 2008). Yet, the examination of a range of healthcare statistics does not demonstrate greater quality when compared with other industrialized countries (World Health Report 2000). An additional observation is that tens of millions of Americans (47 million in 2008) do not have health insurance. This has meant that when they need non-emergency acute or urgent healthcare, they frequently seek it in hospital emergency rooms, which are expensive providers of non-emergency healthcare. Furthermore, even when they receive care in this manner, they are often unable to afford effective follow-up care. This in turn further increases their morbidity and the need for more intensive care and increases the total cost of medical care for society.

Besides having a diffuse safety net to ensure insurance coverage for its citizens compared with other industrialized countries, the United States has proportionally a far greater number of specialists and fewer primary care physicians. This misalignment of primary care physicians and specialists also adds to the basic cost of delivering quality healthcare for a number of reasons. First, a large portion of a specialist's practice may be in primary care. The cost of a specialist delivering primary care may be greater than that of a primary care doctor treating the same disorder. Second, educational costs are driven up in a training system that can be seen as overeducating many doctors who practise their specialty in only a limited fashion. An additional factor adding to the cost of care is the potential excessive use of technology such as imaging devices to establish diagnoses when many diagnoses could be made by less expensive means (Gawande 2009). For instance, outpatient for-profit MRI imaging centres now flourish throughout the country. All these factors, coupled with a view by many that quality medical care for any disorder can only by delivered by specialists, serve to drive up America's total medical bill.

As the cost of medical care has increased, medical leaders and policy-makers have argued for a need to reform the American healthcare system. As society became concerned about the cost of medical care having an adverse impact on the national economy, organized medicine has until recently remained only an observer. To some it may have appeared that rather than focusing on developing mechanisms to moderate cost increases, organized medicine was more concerned about protecting physician incomes. Restated, organized medicine has been seen by some today to function not as a profession guarding quality healthcare, but as a guild protecting physician income prerogatives. Small groups of doctors have founded organizations to address issues of reform, but they have not generally been in the mainstream of organized medicine. To respond to this perception, the AMA developed a national media campaign in 2008 to address the need to develop programmes to ensure all Americans have access to quality medical care.

Quality healthcare and the Institute of Medicine

In addition to the concerns about the cost of healthcare, there has also been a recent concern regarding its quality. In the 1990s the Institute of Medicine (IOM), a subsidiary of the National Academy of Sciences (NAS), raised a number of concerns regarding the quality of healthcare that Americans receive (Institute of Medicine Reports 1999). Healthcare quality is an area where the concerns of society for the welfare of its citizens intersect with the concern of the medical profession for the quality of care its members provide. The area of quality of care forces society and the profession to address head on a number of critical issues. Does society provide adequate resources for all levels of medical education? Does society provide adequate resources for the competent practice of medicine? Does it appropriately monitor through licensure the quality and competence of practitioners? Are medicine's approaches to monitoring the healthcare delivered by its practitioners adequate? Society is responsible for providing adequate facilities and for providing citizens with adequate insurance or funding so that they will receive quality healthcare. Medicine is responsible for monitoring the standards of medical education and the development of protocols to ensure the sustained competence of physicians to practise medicine.

As discussed earlier, in the early 1900s the AMA, acting on its own initiative and speaking for the medical profession without societal input or concern, raised similar questions (Flexner 1910). The power of that action is still felt in American medicine today. But in the 1990s when the responsibilities for ensuring quality healthcare were diffused between a number of medical organizations, it was not clear which organization should respond and how. Finally, the ACGME took the initiative to explicitly define the competencies that are essential to becoming a physician while in residency training. It was intended that attaining these competencies would enhance their practice of medicine and address issues of quality (Accreditation Council for Graduate Medical Education Outcome Project 1999). The ACGME referred to these as the core or general competencies. Additional competencies are described for each specialty. These competencies describe the basic requirements of being a physician and are one of the elements of medical professionalism.

As noted elsewhere in this volume, the Flexner Report addressed similar aims. The United States had 107 851 residents in 8490 residency programmes (Accreditation Council for Graduate Medical Education 2009). It is ACGME that oversees residency standards.

The ACGME's core competencies are:

- Patient care
- Medical knowledge
- Practice-based learning and improvement
- Systems-based practice
- Professionalism
- Interpersonal and communication skills

(ACGME 1999).

The concept of professionalism stated in the core competency leads to some confusion. It relates most clearly to the moral and ethical standards of practice and the behaviours of physicians. The Hippocratic Oath view of competency as applied to the modern practitioner sees all of the competencies as essential and part of professionalism. The core competencies do not address the physician's responsibilities to society.

Since they were developed by the ACGME, these competencies have become a model for medical school, residency training and post-residency education. The integration of the competencies into medicine compares favourably with the Flexner Report of 1910. The impetus for this reform came from the Institute of Medicine (IOM) and represented governmental or societal concerns. The actual generations of the reform activities and their implementation have been performed by organized medicine.

Consumers and providers

Sometime in the past two decades, new terms have been introduced to describe the once seemingly sacred doctor–patient relationship. These terms are 'consumer' and 'provider'.

Some individuals now refer to themselves as consumers of healthcare and refer to the doctors as the providers. While the terms are descriptively correct, they do not address the relationship between the two. For some this is seen as an improvement. They see the doctor–patient relationship as a paternalistic one, with the doctor telling the patient what they should or should not do. The doctor and patient in this view are unequal. In the consumer–provider model they are equal. The consumer is free to accept or reject the provider's recommendations. Today an individual can, if they wish, use the Internet and obtain the same information that the provider holds regarding their illness and the potential form of treatment. However, even if the patient uses the Internet, the doctor still retains the greater understanding of the clinical information and how best to treat their medical issues.

These changes require alterations in the behaviour of the physician. As always, since Hippocrates the doctor must defer to the autonomy and capacity of the patient to make decisions. Exercising and communicating professional clinical judgements is the responsibility of the physician. The patient is free to accept or reject the doctor's recommendations. The physician must respect the patient's choices. We must not confuse commercial standards of behaviour in addressing our patients with professional standards. Although our patients may disagree with our recommendations, we must maintain a continued focus on their wellbeing. The professional standard of behaviour requires more of the doctor not only in treating the patient, but also in dealing with the public good and their own education.

Professionalism in 2010 and beyond

It is generally agreed that healthcare in the United States in 2010 is in a crisis. In this climate varied groups are arguing for dramatic change. The first change mostly discussed in 2010 involves how to insure the 47 million Americans without health insurance. The recently enacted Health Care Protection and Affordable Care Act of 2010 will reduce this number to 17 million over the next 5 years. Many feel this is still an unacceptable number. Further questions remain as to how to increase efficiency, how to effectively use evolving information technology and how to enhance quality. In responding to the call for reform, organized medicine will have to develop responses which address the public good while concurrently addressing guild issues related to the income of its members. Medical practice may need to be modified while still retaining the core value of the doctor–patient relationship. Society will expect a heightened medical concern about quality care coupled with appropriate actions.

The actions of the ACGME and the lifelong focus on the core competencies will probably reduce the likelihood of government intervention in this area. Perhaps the greatest challenge to medicine will be brought about by the growing public knowledge of medicine and that, although vast medical knowledge can be attained by every citizen through the Internet, a well-trained physician is essential to interpret it.

Training new American doctors in professionalism in the early twenty-first century

For new physicians to practise the tenets of the Hippocratic Oath in the twenty-first century, they must adhere to the requirements of medical professionalism. How should they be trained? Medical students and residents have one and frequently only one major concern. That concern is to master as much medicine as they possibly can in a few years. Some maintain interests in other areas and others become experts on public policy matters. For most the issue can best be seen as to how to provide the best care for their individual patients. In this context lectures and ceremonies on professionalism may have limited long-term impact. We believe senior physicians have two areas that they must aid young physicians in learning. First is to practise medicine at a high-quality level while incorporating the modern tenets of the Hippocratic Oath, and second is to support the broad area of professionalism as medicine relates to society.

Physician mentors are also needed in their clerkships to aid students in addressing the inevitable conflicts doctors must face in delivering care. When they see or believe they have seen breakdowns in the quality of care their patients receive or of ethical standards of practice, they will need faculty who will not be grading their work with whom to address these concerns.

Positive messages are more important than negative ones (see also Chapter 11). We propose that throughout medical school and residency, seminars with invited government leaders or involvement with medical schools or hospital administrators be made a part of the students' and residents' curricula as they deal with government learning about leadership. Interaction with state licensing boards as well as with the workings of the LCME and the ACGME would provide valuable experiences. The exact curricula would be determined by the location and structure of each medical school, but the students and residents must be involved if medicine as a profession is to survive.

Conclusions

We have traced professionalism in American medicine for over the past 100 years. Medicine must apply its evolving knowledge to society as it experiences substantial change. To retain its professional standing as a servant of society, medicine must be attuned to the public good and the evolving needs of its citizens. Clear standards of professional performance must be established, and new procedures must be developed to educate its students and practitioners.

References

Accreditation Council for Graduate Medical Education (1999). *General Competencies.* Outcome Project. www.acgme.org/outcome/comp/compCPRL.asp. Last accessed 25 April 2010.

Accreditation Council for Graduate Medical Education (2009). *Report on Number of Programs 2007–2008.* www.acgme.org/adspublic/reports/accredited_programs.asp?accredited=1. Last accessed 25 April 2010.

American Board of Medical Specialties (2000). *Annual Report.* Evanston: American Board of Medical Specialties.

American Medical Association Archives (2007). *Physician Census.* Chicago: American Medical Association.

American Medical Association Archives (2009). *Physician Membership.* Chicago: American Medical Association.

American Psychiatric Association (2009). *Membership Data.* Arlington: American Psychiatric Association.

Atlanta Journal and Constitution (2009). 16 January 2009, p. 1A.

Centers for Medicare and Medicaid Services (2009). *National Health Expenditure Data – Historical.* www.cms.gov/NationalHealthExpendData/02_NationalHealthAccountsHistorical.asp#TopOfPage. Last accessed 29 April 2010.

Flexner A (1910). *Medical Education in the United States and Canada.* Boston: Merrymount Press.

Gawande A (2009). *The Cost Conundrum.* New York: New Yorker, pp. 36–44.

Institute of Medicine Reports (1999). *To Err Is Human: Building a Safer Health System.* Washington, DC: Institute of Medicine.

Lasagna L (1964). *A Modern Version of the Hippocratic Oath.* www.pbs.org/wgbh/nova/doctors/Oath_mopdern.html. Last accessed 25 April 2010.

Liaison Committee on Medical Education (2009). www.lcme.org. Last accessed 20 April 2010.

Ludwig E (1943). *The Hippocratic Oath: Text, Translation, and Interpretation.* Baltimore: Johns Hopkins Press.

National Resident Matching Program (2009). *Match Results 2009.* Washington, DC: National Resident Matching Program.

The Patient Protection and Affordable Care Act (2010). http://dpc.senate.gov/dpcdoc-sen healthcarebill.cfm. Last accessed 4 June 2010.

The World Health Report (2000). *World Health Organization's Ranking of the World's Health Systems.* www.photius.com/rankings/healthranks.html. Last accessed 25 April 2010.

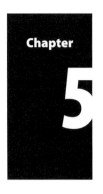

Chapter 5

Professionalism
The UK perspective

Sir Donald Irvine, Neil Johnson, Jill Thistlethwaite and Gillian Lewando Hundt

Editors' introduction

In the past two decades, a run of highly publicized medical scandals in the UK have affected the reputation of the medical profession. Beginning with Bristol, it was the cumulative effect of several such scandals, coming in quick succession, which fired up the public. Together they had a huge impact on the public mind, with the result that public opinion demanded that doctors be regulated more stringently. Consequently, the regulatory body, the General Medical Council (GMC), found its role came under increased scrutiny. The medical royal colleges decided to look at the role of doctors in various settings.

Irvine *et al.* address the need for redefining professionalism, particularly in the context of regulation and continuing professional development. Using *Good Medical Practice* as described by the GMC as the basis of their discussion of professionalism, the authors suggest that the fundamental principle for an individual doctor is about their conscience and knowing what is right. Individually and collectively, team members have to ensure that patients and their carers get the right information, have autonomy and are respected. Thus, there is a collective professional conscience as well. Regulatory and professional bodies have a duty to ensure that these standards are disseminated, acknowledged, reached and maintained. Taking a historical perspective, Irvine *et al.* point out that changes in knowledge lead to changes in skills and required competencies which contribute to the redefinition of professionalism. Professionalism does not occur in a vacuum and has to be seen in the appropriate medical and cultural context.

Introduction

Ideally, when illness strikes, people want doctors who are clinically excellent and who are able and willing to relate to them, respect them and care for them well (Irvine 2007). Patients know that what their doctor does can make the difference between life or death, between enjoying a full recovery or suffering serious disability, and between being treated as a disease or cared for as a person. No-one in their right mind deliberately looks for a careless doctor – they may well have enough to worry about without also having to wonder about their doctor's clinical ability and attitude. This is why patients want doctors they can trust, without even having to think about it. When they say that their doctor is 'very professional', that is what they mean. Thus, in this sense, it is 'professionalism' that is the very essence of being a good doctor.

Professionalism in Mental Healthcare: Experts, Expertise and Expectations, ed. Dinesh Bhugra and Amit Malik. Published by Cambridge University Press. © Cambridge University Press 2011.

In this chapter, we begin by considering what constitutes professionalism in medicine. We then look at the recent history of medical professionalism in the UK and conclude that, whilst we have reached a position in which the regulatory framework is modern and potentially robust, there is still much to be done to ensure that professionalism is embedded deep within every doctor, part of their identity. Education is key to achieving this, so we close by considering the priorities on which we believe those involved in medical education should concentrate.

What is medical professionalism?

The terms 'medical professionalism' and 'profession' continue to be the subject of lively discussion and debate, in particular regarding what the attributes of professionalism are.

In 2004, Cruess *et al.* proposed an adaptation for medicine of the general definition of professions given in the *Oxford English Dictionary* (OED 1989). They described the medical profession as

an occupation whose core element is work based upon a mastery of a complex body of knowledge and skills. It is a vocation in which some department of science or learning or the practice of an art founded upon it is used in the service of others. Its members are governed by codes of ethics and profess a commitment to competence, integrity and morality, altruism, and the promotion of the public good within their domain. These commitments form the basis of a social contract between a profession and society, which in turn grants the profession a monopoly over the use of its knowledge base, the right to considerable autonomy in practice, and the privilege of self-regulation. Professions and their members are accountable to those served, to the profession, and to society. (p. 75)

Whilst this describes the features of professions within society, recent studies (e.g. Wensing *et al.* 1998, Coulter 2005, Bendapudi 2006, Chisholm *et al.* 2006, Hasman *et al.* 2006) have related professionalism to the public's expectations of doctors. Patients and their families think of a good doctor in terms of up-to-date medical knowledge and clinical skill, clinical experience, sound judgement, wisdom, reliability, thoroughness, honesty and general integrity. Good doctors are respectful, kind, courteous, considerate, empathetic and caring. They are interested in their patients, listen to them, are able to communicate effectively, and thus are able to form a satisfactory relationship with them. They go out of their way to explore their patients' feelings, fears, beliefs, values and preferences. Instinctively they put their patients' interests first, making them feel special.

The Royal College of Physicians combined the expectations of patients and doctors by defining professionalism in 2005 as 'a set of values, behaviours and relationships that underpin the trust the public has in doctors' (RCP 2005, p. 14). Controversially, the College argued for abandoning notions of mastery, autonomy, privilege and self-regulation. On the other hand, they said there were self-evident grounds for keeping notions of knowledge, skills, science, profession, society, service, commitment and integrity. Altruism caused real problems. In the event the College decided to retain altruism but qualified its position by recalling that, amongst many doctors, commitment to excellence at work had to be reconciled with the needs of the professional in terms of the latter's own self-care and wellbeing.

Irvine (1997a) and Hafferty (2006) summarized the wide range of descriptors of professionalism. Irvine described medical professionalism as 'resting on three pillars – expertise, ethics and service' (1997a, p. 1540). Expertise derives from a body of knowledge and skills whose utility is constantly invigorated by the results of research. Ethical behaviour flows from a unique combination of values and standards. Service embodies a vocational commitment to put patients first. Similarly, Hafferty (2006) settled for a tripartite framework of core knowledge and skills, ethical principles and selfless and/or service orientation.

These definitions, along with the insights offered by the Picker Institute Europe (Askham and Chisholm 2006, Askham *et al.* 2008) and the Kings Fund (Rosen and Dewar 2004), have made substantial contributions to rethinking professionalism in recent years and are affecting the wider reforms of professional regulation led by the GMC, the medical royal colleges and the government.

The key thing for British doctors is that, whatever individual writers say, the attributes of professionalism that they are now expected to demonstrate in daily practice are those described by the GMC in *Good Medical Practice* (GMC 2006a) and its accompanying guidance on specific ethical topics. The characteristics of the 'good doctor' are all reflected in that code of practice.

There is a further fundamental point to make here. For the individual doctor, professionalism should be essentially about conscience, about reflecting and being motivated to act on an inner conviction about what is 'right' for that person. But there is a collective component to such personal conviction. Groups of individuals (e.g. clinical teams, professional bodies, National Health Service (NHS) organizations) work together for the benefit of those who use the service. Collectively, as well as individually, members have a duty to ensure that patients and their families are safe, involved in healthcare decisions, well informed and treated with respect; this duty also involves ensuring that other members of staff are treated with respect, their views listened to and their concerns taken seriously. Thus, professionalism is about collective conscience as well as personal conviction – they are two sides of the same coin. In medicine, it is important that the profession's standards bodies, including the GMC, royal colleges and professional societies, should acknowledge, lead and act on this collective conscience.

There is a risk that, if professionalism is not based on a combination of personal conviction and collective conscience, it will be seen purely in terms of compliance with externally imposed regulations – 'ticking the box'. In turn, this may result in minds and behaviours that focus on 'just getting by'. In contrast, practitioners who are strongly motivated to do the right thing are more likely to strive for excellence. Self-evidently, the stronger the inner conviction in individual doctors, the more likely it is that patients will be assured of sustained excellence; similarly, the more doctors there are who can demonstrate that they share such conviction, the stronger and more coherent the collective profession will become. In our view it is therefore essential that attention be paid to the development of personal conviction *and* collective conscience, and we will return to this theme when considering the role of medical education.

The evolution of medical professionalism in the UK

During the past century, medical practice changed out of all recognition. As Sir Cyril Chantler (1999) said, 'medicine used to be simple, ineffective and relatively safe. Now it is complex, effective and potentially dangerous' (p. 1181). In little more than a century, unprecedented advances in medical science have changed the nature and mode of medical practice, and with it the organization and management of healthcare.

Equally dramatically, society itself has changed. We live in a consumer world in which the practice of medicine has been demystified. The public no longer has to rely on doctors for information about medical matters because people have independent access to the database of medicine through the Internet. That fact, and the emergence of patient autonomy, has altered the dynamics of the patient–doctor relationship decisively in favour of the patient. Consequently, more patients want an open relationship with their doctors. They want to be well informed and involved in decisions about their care (Gertais *et al.* 1993, Coulter 2005, Chisholm *et al.* 2006).

So, professionalism cannot be seen as a free-standing entity. It has to be seen in context (Irvine 1997a, Hafferty 2006), in tune with the state of healthcare and the social conditions and expectations of the time. In this brief review of the history of professional regulation, we will concentrate on two aspects: first, the development of the regulatory framework which now exists; and second, the role of collective professionalism in achieving this.

Earlier times: 1858–1989

British doctors gained state recognition as professionals in 1858 with the passing of the first Medical Act and the formation of the GMC to implement it on Parliament's behalf. The Act accorded doctors huge privileges, such as control over entry to the profession, their education and, through this, the content of their work, and permission to regulate themselves (self-regulation), as well as enhanced social status and income.

Between 1858 and the end of the 1980s, doctors generally assumed that professionalism and membership of the profession were one and the same thing (Fox 1951, Stacey 1992, Irvine 2003). Professional values, protective of patients and of altruistic service, were grounded on the Hippocratic Oath; it was assumed that doctors would absorb and internalize them. As a corollary, professional 'misconduct' was very unlikely to concern the average reasonably conscientious doctor as it was largely about criminal behaviour, sexual misconduct with patients or breaches of patient confidentiality. The avoidance of breaches of professional etiquette (designed to protect doctors' own interests) such as advertising, taking another doctor's patients or criticizing a colleague's clinical practice – 'there but for the grace of God go I' – was more likely to be in doctors' minds in their everyday work.

In 1948 the Labour government founded the NHS. Paternalistic professionalism was the order of the day, and this was reinforced unwittingly in the early years of the NHS by politicians who quickly realized that there would have to be some form of rationing. They knew that at that time they were less powerful than the doctors and that the public would not trust them with this responsibility. So the obvious answer was to get the doctors, whom the public did trust, to do the job for them. The state and professional leaders reached an informal understanding, the implicit 'social contract', that reinforced medicine's virtually total control over standards, education and governance in exchange for doctors' willingness to ration access to expensive healthcare, most clearly demonstrated through the control of waiting lists via the GP referral system (Irvine 2003, p. 29).

Stability was the order of the day until the early seventies when, as a result of doctors' anger about their lack of adequate representation on the GMC, a parliamentary inquiry (The Merrison Inquiry 1972–1975) was held into the regulation of the medical profession. The Inquiry (Secretary of State for Social Services 1975) gave doctors more say but, from the public's point of view, there was no substantial change. In particular, nothing was done by the Inquiry to address the evidence it had received about the persistence of poor standards of practice (e.g. RCGP 1974), which the GMC had shown no inclination to pursue and indeed had no powers to manage even if it wanted to.

Nevertheless, some of the profession's leaders were uneasy – they knew that the public was not being adequately protected. Immediately after Merrison, they initiated the first tentative attempt to address doctors' ongoing competence to practise. A committee, chaired by Sir Anthony Alment (Committee of Enquiry 1976), considered recertification but concluded that it would be unacceptable to doctors and anyway would be too difficult to implement. So nothing happened, although the committee did note that 'in today's fast moving society .... a plea for protection from control mechanisms for a selected group of individuals who possess knowledge and skills of importance to the general public may well seem to be a case of special pleading' (p. 46).

But times were changing. The earlier stable social contract between profession and state was coming under pressure. The 1980s saw the rise of managerialism and commercialism in the NHS, 'the blitzkrieg from the right' as Sir Maurice Shock described it (Shock 1994), as successive governments struggled to contain costs and bring more accountability to health professionals' practice. Similarly, with what the late Professor Meg Stacey called 'the Patients' Revolt' (Stacey 1992), important non-medical voices, albeit still few in number, were now beginning to be raised about the GMC's – and therefore the profession's – attitudes to patients, and particularly to poor practice. For example, Professor Ian Kennedy (Kennedy 1983), in his 1981 Reith lectures on the *Unmasking of Medicine*, wanted regular re-registration (now called revalidation), a 'Code of Professional Standards of Competence', an Inspectorate and a sensitive complaints procedure to maintain good practice and deal with questionable practice. In 1983 Rudolf Klein, Professor of Social Policy at Bath University, focused on doctors' accountability and the way in which the GMC confined itself to extreme cases of misconduct whilst ignoring indifferent practice (Klein 1983). In 1988 Mrs Jean Robinson, working for the Patients' Association and a lay member of the GMC, published a devastating critique of the GMC's performance in dealing with transparency and poor practice (Robinson 1988). Meanwhile, in 1989 the British Medical Journal published a series of nine papers by assistant editor Richard Smith that were highly critical of the GMC (Smith 1989).

Stacey (1992), in an insightful analysis of the history of UK professional self-regulation through the GMC and the current fitness for purpose of the GMC, summed up the attitude of both the profession and the GMC towards the protection of the public thus:

The problem was to understand how it could be that essentially decent and well meaning men (mostly men) of high ethical standards could operate a system which colluded in the maintenance of an outdated educational system and served the public so ill in matters of discipline and confidence. (p. 27)

It was by now clear that the traditional approach to professionalism and reactive self-regulation had been found wanting. The social contract between public and profession was breaking down.

Out with the old, in with the new: 1990–2009

In 1990 the GMC embarked on three new developments. In 1992 it published *Tomorrow's Doctors*, a radical shake-up of medical education (GMC 1992). In 1995, in a fundamental break with the past, it published a new code of practice, *Good Medical Practice* (GMC 1995), and that same year, following a change it had secured to the Medical Act, it began work on the implementation of its new performance procedures.

The profession was then further shaken by the disclosure of the failures in paediatric cardiac surgery at the Bristol Royal Infirmary (Bristol Royal Infirmary Inquiry 2001). In 1998, two surgeons and the medically qualified chief executive of the hospital were found guilty by the GMC of serious professional misconduct (GMC 1998). Day after day, the hearing had put the state of professional regulation on the front page of every newspaper. Several other cases – Ledward, Shipman and Neale – reinforced the picture of a profession, a GMC and an NHS that had all been casual about poor practice. It was Bristol and these other cases that impelled radical changes, not only in medical regulation, but also by putting the many aspects of healthcare quality and patient safety seriously onto the NHS agenda for the first time. Therefore, between 1998 and 2001, the GMC laid the foundations for the strengthened model of professional regulation described below (Irvine 1997b).

However, not all doctors accepted all aspects of reform without challenge. The focal point of professional opposition was revalidation, i.e. the proposed regular review of the performance of doctors, because it required a new order of professionalism and accountability from every doctor (GMC 2000). The battle between reforming doctors and conservative doctors was bitter (Irvine 2003). To rebuild public trust, the reformers essentially wanted a regular, robustly evidence-based evaluation of all doctors' practice, with public participation in the assessment process and external scrutiny, whilst the conservatives, acknowledging that there would have to be some form of process, wanted the minimum consistent with good appearances.

Dame Janet Smith highlighted this division in her report on the Shipman Inquiry (The Shipman Inquiry 2004). She held a mirror up to the GMC's policies and procedures, particularly its plans for revalidation and fitness to practise. In her in-depth examination of the GMC's role (pp. 1023–1176), she indicated that she had been prepared to accept the proposals for revalidation and fitness to practise in their original robust form as evidence that the GMC had put the past behind it. However, in later changes designed to placate the conservatives, the GMC had apparently reverted to its old ways, accommodating professional self-interest on the basis of 'expediency' not 'principle' (Smith 2004). Dame Janet found these later proposals inconsistent with the GMC's declared aim of adequately protecting the public.

It was this critical report and the subsequent review by the Chief Medical Officer, Sir Liam Donaldson, that it precipitated, which finally stimulated the changes in professional regulation now being implemented (Donaldson 2006).

The new professionalism

The new model of professionalism, advanced by the GMC and others, has four main elements: the foundation, the standards themselves; compliance mechanisms mainly through regulation and contracts of service; the responsibility for internalizing the professional standards primarily through medical education; and the moral obligation on professional institutions to uphold collective professionalism. These fundamental changes, together with much more public involvement in the GMC itself, are intended to signal a decisive break with the doctor-centric professionalism of the past, putting patients' interests unequivocally first. As Freidson (2001) wrote, professional codes of practice are 'mere rhetoric if they are not rigorously (though sensitively) enforced … If professionalism is to be reasserted and regain some of its influence, it must elaborate and refine its code of ethics but also strengthen their methods of adjudicating and correcting their violation' (p. 215).

Good Medical Practice (GMC 2006a) sets out the generic principles, values and duties on which good practice is founded. Versions containing additional, specialty-specific standards have been produced by each of the medical royal colleges. For example, *Good Psychiatric Practice* describes the standards expected of psychiatrists (Royal College of Psychiatrists 2009). *Good Medical Practice* is therefore the basis of licensure, certification and revalidation

Table 5.1 Summary of current regulatory framework

Licensure	From 2009 the GMC will issue licences to practise as a doctor. The privileges and responsibilities previously associated with registration will be transferred to the new licence. Initial licensure signifies the satisfactory completion of basic medical education.
Certification	Alongside their licence, doctors practising in any recognized specialty will need to have the necessary Certificate of Completion of Training.
Revalidation	Revalidation, combining relicensure by the GMC and complementary recertification by the Royal Colleges, will be the process through which doctors will be required to demonstrate regularly that they are fit to practise in their chosen field.
Fitness to practise	The GMC retains the power to review a doctor's fitness to continue to practise and to remove a doctor's licence.

and informs the whole of medical education.[1] The GMC states that the code describes medical professionalism in action. It provides clear and accessible standards related to everyday professional practice. It embodies patients' expectations through the incorporation of evidence-based research conducted for the GMC by the Picker Institute (Chisholm *et al.* 2006). It gives patients a benchmark against which to judge their experiences, and it tells doctors explicitly that serious or persistent failure to follow the guidance will put their registration at risk.

The approach to regulation taken by the GMC now involves four components, which are summarized in Table 5.1.

Collective professionalism

Within the medical profession, the royal colleges and faculties, and many professional societies, are the main source of expertise in their field. Therefore, we would argue, they have a special responsibility to give leadership on standards of professionalism in their respective specialties. Two examples, one old and one new, illustrate the point.

In the late 1940s, general practice was in a mess. In a famous study, Joseph Collings (1950) described huge variations in the quality of practice, with much that was truly awful. A small number of conscientious doctors who cared about their patients and the good name of their branch of medicine accepted responsibility for these failings. Together they founded the College of General Practitioners (now the RCGP) in 1952. Over the next 20 years they set about introducing standards for practice and proper training where previously there had been none, and establishing an evidence base for the discipline. They were the first to look outside medicine for inspiration, using insights from social scientists, educationalists, patients and other professions with different views of medicine, and in doing so introduced a foretaste of the kind of thinking about professionalism that would come to the rest of medicine later. They transformed ideas about general practice.

The second example is drawn from cardiac surgery today. We have already mentioned the disaster at Bristol. What happened subsequently is that the UK Society for Cardiothoracic Surgery, led by Sir Bruce Keogh, set about rebuilding their specialty around a new national database (Bridgewater *et al.* 2009), with the public reporting of individual surgeons' survival rates as a central principle. In doing so, they have set a new and higher standard of

---

[1] Registration, stripped of practising privileges, will be reserved for non-practising doctors who nevertheless want to maintain their demonstrable commitment to the ethical duties and obligations of the profession set out in *Good Medical Practice*.

professionalism, offering inspiration to other branches of medicine and gaining a deepened sense of trust from patients.

These two examples, separated in time, have three vital characteristics. First, they were both born of a realization from within that the status quo was unacceptable, that something had to be done and that the relevant professionals had to take the initiative themselves. Second, remarkable individuals came forward to give determined professional leadership, especially when confronted with scepticism or even downright hostility from those opposed to change. And third, a determination to succeed in the face of adversity resulted in a strong sense of esprit, a high overall standard of performance and high morale across the two groups as a whole.

Professionalism at the workplace

Two recent developments are likely to influence attitudes to professionalism at work. The first is clinical governance and the opportunities that it should afford in future for the regular peer review of practice. Annual formative and summative appraisal will be at the heart of this, informed by multisource feedback complementing other performance data available for revalidation and recertification. As an incentive to high performance, we would support a strong track record of professionalism as a contributory requirement for clinical excellence awards in future.

The second development will be in the routine use of near virtual feedback of patients' experience of all clinicians, including individual doctors. The Picker Institute envisages that this powerful new tool has the potential to transform doctors' understanding of their actual relationship with patients in the near future, particularly if the results are made public.

Medical education and professionalism

We concluded earlier that professionalism is dependent on developing inner conviction and collective conscience. Without this deep internalization, there is a major risk that doctors will equate professionalism with merely doing 'enough' to ensure that they are not 'caught out'. The initial development and subsequent maintenance of professional standards is the role of medical education.

There are three main phases. Basic medical education involves that period up to the point of graduation from medical school. The GMC regulates this phase against the standards set out in *Tomorrow's Doctors*. Postgraduate medical education (including the generic period of foundation training and later periods of specialty training) is managed by postgraduate medical deaneries against the standards set by the relevant royal colleges (or UK Foundation Programme); it is currently regulated by the Postgraduate Medical Education and Training Board (PMETB), which will be incorporated within the GMC by 2010. Education beyond the completion of postgraduate training is based on 'continuing professional development' (CPD). The introduction of appraisal and revalidation will bring the CPD phase also within the regulatory framework of the GMC and the colleges.

As a first step to internalization, it is crucial that those entering medicine understand exactly what professionalism and the associated code of practice represent. First, it is important to acknowledge explicitly that professionalism relates to every aspect of the work of a doctor. It *is* about the total identity of the doctor, about a way of working in all aspects of care – putting patients first, ensuring the highest standards of care, maintaining one's own and others' practice and working very effectively with colleagues to achieve that. It is *not* simply a set of regulations to be learnt once and then referred to when decisions have to be made at the boundaries of the code (e.g. decisions about what constitutes euthanasia or when it is acceptable for a doctor to break confidentiality). Second, and as a direct corollary, those becoming doctors need to appreciate that the rationale behind having a written code of practice is to provide all doctors with a common framework within which they practise, rather than an attempt to control their every move. It is about sharing the same standards, not about trying to mould personalities to be the same.

Furthermore, to achieve this deep embedding, it is essential that those who lead, manage and regulate medical education address those aspects of the curriculum that are hidden and/or informal with as much vigour as they do for those aspects that are overt (Hafferty and Franks 1994). Thus, in its design and delivery, the curriculum should not only ensure that all elements of professionalism are addressed with appropriate balance between the elements, but should also acknowledge and make use of the informal and hidden just as much as the overt. To do this we emphasize four aspects of the curriculum.

Recognition and use of the power of modelling

Future doctors are strongly influenced by the models of practice they observe (Cruess *et al.* 2008). This has three significant implications.

At the individual level, all those who have a role in teaching or supervising must actively model those values we are encouraging future doctors to internalize – that is, the teacher should not only model the values but should also make explicit how these values are being used to shape decisions. This is particularly important when a decision or behaviour by the supervisor or teacher might appear counter-intuitive. In the UK, the introduction of regular appraisal as part of revalidation will undoubtedly cause medical teachers (and their employing institutions) to reflect continuously on their standards of professional practice and the ways in which they make this overt to those in training.

At the collective level, within those organizations that provide, manage and regulate education, there must be a culture that enables and ensures that everyone within the organization models these values. For example, medical students and trainee doctors are able to evaluate the behaviour of their tutors, clinical teachers and peers but are often unsure of how to influence these behaviours. If the organization does not allow suboptimal behaviour to be challenged, the junior members of the hierarchy become disillusioned and ignore further examples, or even start to mirror the behaviours themselves. Similarly, just as the curriculum will explicitly emphasize the importance of developing doctors' abilities to listen effectively to patients, new doctors need to experience being heard effectively themselves. This is a significant challenge in medical education as there is no single organization with sole responsibility for education. This means that organizations must work collectively to ensure that these values are upheld throughout the education system. Fortunately, the development of such a culture will have wider positive consequences, as we know that organizations with a culture of honesty and responsiveness to constructive and timely feedback enhance patient safety (Runciman *et al.* 2007).

As a corollary, all those involved in medical education must demonstrate collective professionalism. Just as the profession should take responsibility for leading system-wide change in healthcare, those responsible for medical education must take collective responsibility for leading change in medical education.

The final implication is that if health professionals are to work together effectively they need to learn together. This does raise a tension as professional codes and ways of working vary across professions. However, whilst the code of conduct is not exactly the same for all healthcare professions (an issue that can lead to poor communication and misunderstanding), the areas of commonality between codes of conduct are much greater than the differences.

Involvement of patients in teaching and assessment

Promoting patient-centred learning through the involvement of patients and carers in teaching and assessment is another strategy for developing professionalism. Patients have always been vital in helping students learn the clinical skills of history taking, physical examination and clinical diagnosis. However, in the past decade their role within the curricula of medical schools has broadened, with an emphasis on active participation and roles beyond the clinical placement (BMA 2008). For example, in many medical school curricula, students visit families in their homes and learn about the impact of illness on their lives. Families involved in one such course reported that they participate in this so that the students will become doctors who will listen to patients in future (Jackson *et al.* 2003). The GMC is keen to encourage active patient and public involvement in medical education and indeed applaud it when they find it (GMC Quality Assurance Report on Warwick Medical School 2006b, para. 126). However, there is no specific financial resource for patient involvement. This contrasts with social care education, where there is ring-fenced funding for every social work course for the development and practice of user involvement in teaching provision.

Guidance on mechanisms and best practice in this field are scarce, and there is significant current debate about the best ways to develop this aspect of the curriculum. Users and carers can be involved in classroom-based and clinical teaching, assessment and admissions, and in curriculum development at all levels. It is, however, vital in our view that we put mechanisms in place to support the professional development of service users and carers, with clear guidelines regarding payment and their remit. This is an emergent area within medical education, but we believe that it is pivotal in the development of patient-centred education and care and, therefore, of professionalism.

Attention to the dilemmas faced by those early in their careers

Experienced clinicians recognize that upholding high standards of professionalism on a daily basis constantly raises dilemmas. Doctors early in their careers have less personal experience on which to draw. Therefore, it is essential that trainees have the chance to discuss the dilemmas they face and explore how they might be resolved. Tensions will arise when an individual's values are at odds with those of the profession or society. For example, for the nurse who feels that abortion is wrong or the doctor who believes that euthanasia is acceptable, to what extent should collective conscience overrule personal conviction? Similarly, in day-to-day practice, what is the appropriate balance between the needs of patients and the personal needs of the professional, how far should self-care be taken, and might this be mistaken for neglecting responsibility? Doctors in training need to have opportunities to consider their responses to these dilemmas. We would strongly advocate that these opportunities should allow them to draw on the reflections of experienced colleagues and of patients too.

Explicit assessment of professionalism

Although there are increasing attempts to assess professionalism (e.g. Arnold 2002, Epstein and Hundert 2002, Lynch *et al.* 2004, Veloski *et al.* 2005, Jha *et al.* 2007), assessment remains difficult because there are no agreed criteria nor any widely accepted methods for collecting the necessary evidence. We believe that it is important to address this and suggest that the following principles are used. Given that professionalism is multifaceted, multiple forms of evidence collected on a variety of occasions using observations from a number of sources are necessary. Sources should include patients and colleagues. The types of evidence should be blueprinted against all components of professionalism to ensure that a holistic view is obtained.

Continuing professional development

However, whilst we can apply the four above approaches without great difficulty in basic and postgraduate medical education where the curricula are clearly defined, different methods will be needed for CPD as the curriculum is much more personal. As a first step, CPD must be taken seriously by both individual doctors and their employers; the introduction of revalidation with its continued focus on appraisal will be of significant help in this. As most doctors do perform well much of the time, there is a risk that CPD focused on professionalism may be perceived as criticism, resulting in defensive behaviours such as denial or token involvement. To address this we believe it is important to start from a positive position, with an emphasis on CPD and revalidation as being clearly designed to support doctors. Finally, CPD must address *all* aspects of professionalism – it should no longer be acceptable for doctors to focus solely on one aspect of their development, such as updating their clinical knowledge.

Conclusions and challenges

British medicine is at a crossroads. The decisions of British doctors now will determine the medical profession's trustworthiness and standing with the public and patients in the years ahead. We have no doubt that the cultural revolution now in progress in British medicine will result in much stronger patient-centred professionalism and self-regulation. This will be immensely reassuring to the public and patients and will appeal to the great majority of conscientious doctors who take pride in the standing of their profession.

We conclude that:

- The public should be able to take for granted that all doctors will uphold high standards of care. Everyone is entitled to a good doctor.
- These high standards must be based on a set of values held deep in the individual and collective conscience.
- Doctors themselves have the power and influence to achieve all that we have described in this chapter – but they must take positive collective action to do so, not simply expect it to happen.
- By working together, e.g through the colleges, we should ensure that we uphold the highest standards of professionalism and that the right changes happen. We can achieve this by:
  - Taking responsibility for our profession
  - Leading change rather than expecting others to lead

- Establishing the cultural norms that enable professionalism to develop
- Making sure that patients' experience of care is always as good as possible, and never a cause for worry or concern
- Placing particular emphasis on supporting those who lead the education and development of the next generation.

As doctors, our understanding of the new relationship with our patients and the public finds its outward expression in the values and standards of the new medical culture – the new professionalism.

References

Arnold L (2002). Assessing professional behavior: yesterday, today, and tomorrow. *Academic Medicine* **77**, 502–515.

Askham J, Chisholm A (2006). *Patient-centred Medical Professionalism: Towards an Agenda for Research and Action*. www.pickereurope. org/Filestore/PIE_reports/PCP/ pcpconcepts-report-PDF.pdf. Last accessed 9 March 2010.

Askham J, Chisholm A, Claridge S, Coulter A, Irvine D H, Magee H (2008). *Doctors and Patient-centred Practice*. www.pickereurope. org/Filestore/PIE_reports/project_reports/ PCPfinalreportPIIMay2008.pdf. Last accessed 18 April 2010.

Bendapudi N M, Berry L L, Frey K A, Parish J T, Rayburn W L (2006). Patient perspectives on ideal physician behaviours. *Mayo Clinic Proceedings* **81**, 338–344.

Bridgewater B, Keogh B, Kinsman R, Walton P (2009). *The Society for Cardiothoracic Surgery in GB and Ireland 6th National Database Report: Demonstrating Quality*. London: Dendrite Clinical Systems.

Bristol Royal Infirmary Inquiry (2001). *Learning from Bristol: The Report of the Public Inquiry into Children's Heart Surgery at the Bristol Royal Infirmary 1984–1995*. London: Stationery Office.

British Medical Association (2008). *The Role of the Patient in Medical Education*. London: British Medical Association.

Chantler C (1999). The role and education of doctors in the delivery of health care. *Lancet* **353**, 1178–1181.

Chisholm A, Cairncross I, Askham J (2006). *Setting Standards: The Views of Members of the Public and Doctors on the Standards of Care they Expect from Doctors*. Oxford: Picker Institute Europe. www.pickereurope. org/Filestore/Publications/Setting_ Standards_Finalpdf. Last accessed May 2009.

Collings J S (1950). General practice in England today: a reconnaissance. *Lancet* **1**, 555–585.

Coulter A (2005). What do patients want from primary care? *British Medical Journal* **331**, 1199–2001.

Cruess S R, Cruess R L, Steinert Y (2008). Role modelling – making the most of a powerful teaching strategy. *British Medical Journal* **336**, 718–721.

Cruess S R, Johnston S, Cruess R L (2004). Professionalism: a working definition for medical educators. *Teaching and Learning in Medicine* **16**, 74–76.

Donaldson L (2006). *Good Doctors, Safer Patients*. London: Department of Health.

Epstein R M, Hundert E M (2002). Defining and assessing professional competence. *Journal of the American Medical Association* **287**, 226–235.

Fox T F (1951). Professional freedom. *Lancet* **2**(6673), 115–119.

Freidson E (2001). *Professionalism: The Third Logic*. Cambridge: Polity Press.

General Medical Council (1992). *Tomorrow's Doctors*. London: GMC.

General Medical Council (1995). *Good Medical Practice* (1st edn). London: GMC.

General Medical Council Professional Conduct Committee (1998). Transcript of Proceedings, 17–18 June.

General Medical Council (2000). *Revalidating Doctors: Ensuring Standards, Securing the Future*. London: GMC.

General Medical Council (2006a). *Good Medical Practice* (4th edn). London: GMC.

General Medical Council (2006b). *Quality Assurance Report on Warwick Medical School*. www.gmc.org.uk/education/undergraduate_ qa/reports/warwick_2006. Last accessed 15 June 2009.

Gertais M, Edgman-Levitan S, Daley J, Delbanco TL (eds.) (1993). *Through the Patient's Eyes: Understanding and Promoting Patient-Centred Care*. San Francisco: Jossey-Bass.

Hafferty F W (2006). Definitions of professionalism – a search for meaning and identity. *Clinical Orthopaedics and Related Research* **449**, 193–204.

Hafferty F W, Franks R (1994). The hidden curriculum, ethics teaching, and the structure of medical education. *Academic Medicine* **69**, 861–871.

Hasman A, Graham C, Reeve R, Askham J (2006). *What Do Patients and Relatives See as Key Competencies for Intensive Care Doctors?* Oxford: Picker Institute Europe. www.pickereurope.org/Filestore/Publications/CobatriceFull_report_with isbn_web_(2).pdf. Last accessed 3 May 2009.

Irvine D H (1997a). The performance of doctors. I Professionalism and self-regulation in a changing world. *British Medical Journal* **314**, 1540–1542.

Irvine D H (1997b). The performance of doctors. II: Maintaining good practice: protecting patients from poor performance. *British Medical Journal* **314**, 1613–1615.

Irvine D H (2003). *The Doctor's Tale: Professionalism and Public Trust.* Oxford: Radcliffe Medical Press.

Irvine D H (2007). Everyone is entitled to a good doctor. *Medical Journal of Australia* **186**(5), 256–261.

Jackson A, Blaxter L, Lewando Hundt G (2003). Participating in medical education: views of patients and carers living in deprived communities. *Medical Education* **37**, 1–7.

Jha V, Bekker H L, Duffy S R G, Roberts T E (2007). A systematic review of studies assessing and facilitating attitudes towards professionalism in medicine. *Medical Education* **41**, 822–829.

Kennedy I (1983). *The Unmasking of Medicine.* London: Granada.

Klein R (1983). *The Politics of the National Health Service.* London: Longman.

Lynch D C, Surdyk P M, Eiser A R (2004). Assessing professionalism: a review of the literature. *Medical Teacher* **26**, 366–373.

Oxford English Dictionary (1989). (2nd edn). Oxford: Clarendon Press.

Report of the Committee of Enquiry set up for the medical profession in the United Kingdom (1976). *Competence to Practise.* Chairman Sir Anthony Alment. London: Committee of Enquiry.

Robinson J A (1988). *A Patient's Voice at the GMC: A Lay Member's View of the General Medical Council.* London: Health Rights.

Rosen R, Dewar S (2004). *On Being a Doctor: Redefining Medical Professionalism for Better Patient Care.* London: Kings Fund.

Royal College of General Practitioners (1974). Evidence to the inquiry into the regulation of the medical profession. *Journal of the Royal College of General Practitioners* **24**, 59–74.

Royal College of Physicians (2005). *Doctors in Society: Medical Professionalism in a Changing World. Report of a Working Party.* London: Royal College of Physicians.

Royal College of Psychiatrists (2009). *Good Psychiatric Practice* (3rd edn). London: Royal College of Psychiatrists.

Runciman B, Merryweather A, Walton M (2007). *Safety and Ethics in Healthcare.* Aldershot: Ashgate.

Secretary of State for Social Services (1975). *Report of the Committee of Inquiry into the Regulation of the Medical Profession.* Chairman Dr A W Merrison. Cmnd 6018. London: Stationery Office.

Shock M (1994). Medicine at the centre of the nation's affairs. *British Medical Journal* **309**, 1730–1733.

Smith R (1989). The day of judgement comes closer. *British Medical Journal* **298**, 1241–1244.

Smith R (2004). The GMC: expediency before principle. *British Medical Journal* **330**, 1–2.

Stacey M (1992). *Regulating British Medicine: the General Medical Council.* Chichester: Wiley.

The Shipman Inquiry (2004). *Safeguarding Patients: Lessons from the Past, Proposals for the Future.* Chairman Dame Janet Smith. London: Stationery Office, pp. 1023–1176.

Veloski J J, Fields S K, Boex J R, Blank L L (2005). Measuring professionalism: a review of studies with instruments reported in the literature between 1982 and 2002. *Academic Medicine* **80**, 366–370.

Wensing M, Jung H P, Mainz J, Olesen F, Grol R A (1998). A systematic review of the literature on patient priorities for general practice care. 1. Description of the research domain. *Social Science and Medicine* **47**, 1573–1588.

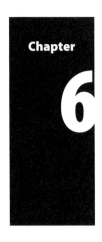

Chapter 6

Professionalism and resource-poor settings
Redefining psychiatry in the context of global mental health

Vikram Patel

Editors' introduction

The Movement for Global Mental Health is a significant step forwards in the delivery of healthcare across the globe. It has particular significance in this era of globalization and extensive migration. The context in which healthcare services are delivered is particularly important in developing mental healthcare. The stigma associated with mental illness and psychiatry takes on different connotations, especially if the cultural explanations of mental illness are related to non-medical causes. In this chapter, Patel argues that in low- and middle-income countries, where resources are limited, the role of the psychiatrist may carry higher levels of non-clinical responsibilities, such as supervision and training, rather than direct clinical contact. Treatment gaps that exist in those countries are further compounded by factors such as a poor agenda for public mental health, complexity of decentralization and challenges related to poor political will in dealing with marginalized individuals with mental illness. Resource disturbance is often tilted in favour of the urban metropolis, and large swathes of rural areas remain uncovered. Patel suggests that, under these circumstances, psychiatrists should be supporting other types of mental healthcare delivery through primary care workers of different specialties. In addition, the role of the psychiatrist should focus on priority research and building capacity through training and supervision. Advocacy as a core function of professionalism in such settings is crucial. The responsibility of the psychiatrist in these settings and situations is also to focus on public mental health.

The treatment gap in mental health

The large 'treatment gap' for people with mental disorders has been well documented in all countries of the world, including those with high levels of resources. However, the gaps are substantially larger in low-income countries and in the resource-poor settings of middle- and high-income countries. Treatment gaps in these contexts approach an astonishing 90%, even for people with serious mental disorders. Thus, it would be fair to conclude that the most common form of care people with mental disorders receive in most parts of the world (and therefore, by extension, most people with mental disorders globally) is home-based

Professionalism in Mental Healthcare: Experts, Expertise and Expectations, ed. Dinesh Bhugra and Amit Malik. Published by Cambridge University Press. © Cambridge University Press 2011.

support from friends and relatives and self-help. Even when people do see help, the quality of this care is mixed. Substantial proportions of people with depressive and anxiety disorders, and substance abuse disorders, who may consult primary care doctors or other primary healthcare practitioners, will receive non-evidence-based interventions; typically, their mental disorders will go unrecognized and they will receive a cocktail of medications for specific symptoms. For example, it is not uncommon for a person with depression in Asia to receive a nutritional supplement or vitamin for fatigue, a hypnotic for insomnia and an analgesic for headache. Psychosocial interventions are very rarely used. Few patients go to specialist services, not least because they are scarce, but also because of the enormous stigma attached to psychiatry in most parts of the world. Specialist care is reserved for people who are severely disabled or disturbed; not surprisingly, earlier authors have argued that psychiatry in developing countries is the 'psychiatry of psychoses'(Asuni 1991) and is for the tiny proportion of relatively affluent and urban populations who have higher levels of 'mental health literacy' and hold less stigmatized views about specialist care. A major reason for stigma is the very nature of specialist care in many countries; much specialist care is concentrated in large mental hospitals, which are sited in locations distant from town centres or from other hospitals, are poorly staffed and inadequately resourced, and where custodial care takes precedence over modern, multimodal interventions designed to facilitate early discharge into a functioning community mental healthcare system (Patel 2009). Human rights abuses, including chaining and beatings, are not uncommon. It is hardly surprising, then, that the vast majority of people with mental disorders do not wish to be associated with psychiatry or psychiatric institutions in most parts of the world.

It is in this sombre context that I consider the need for a radical revision of the professional role of psychiatrists. Although the context for this position is primarily low-income countries (which are, without exception, also very low resourced in mental health services), it may also be true of middle- and high-income countries (and certainly, the resource-poor areas of these countries). I argue that the primary professional role of psychiatrists in these settings is not face-to-face individual clinical encounters; rather, it is a public health role which seeks primarily to close the treatment gap by facilitating steps to scale up services for people with mental disorders according to the twin principles of promoting evidence-based treatments and ensuring the human rights of people with mental disorders and their families. This call for action is the central theme of the Movement for Global Mental Health (www.globalmentalhealth.org), launched on 10 October 2008 (Editorial 2008). At the very least, every psychiatrist can, and should, be a member of this Movement to demonstrate a commitment to these goals.

This chapter will begin by considering the barriers to closing the treatment gaps, focusing primarily on the availability and distribution of specialist human resources. The principal argument arising from this discussion is that the current and forecast numbers of specialists available in most countries are grossly insufficient at present and will never be sufficient to close the treatment gap for the foreseeable future if 'business as usual' continues. The next section will then consider what the alternative roles could comprise to make psychiatry and the other clinical mental health specialist disciplines more relevant and responsive to the vast unmet needs of people with mental disorders globally. For the sake of clarity, I will use the term 'psychiatry' in this chapter to refer to both the medical and other clinical specialties concerned with mental healthcare (notably, psychiatric nursing, clinical psychology and psychiatric social work). The final section will consider the strategies through which psychiatry can, as it were, reinvent itself for the future.

> **Panel 1** Barriers to scaling up services for people with mental disorders (adapted from Saraceno *et al.* 2007)
>
> - The prevailing public health priority agenda and its impact on funding, which typically excludes mental health
> - The complexity of and resistance to decentralizing mental health services
> - The challenges in implementing mental healthcare in primary care settings
> - The limited number and types of human resources trained and supervised in mental healthcare
> - The lack of public health perspectives in mental health leadership.

Barriers to closing the treatment gap

The recent *Lancet* series on global mental health has documented five major barriers to scaling up services for people with mental disorders (Panel 1).

Of all the resource needs in mental healthcare, arguably the greatest one of all is that related to mental health human resources, for the simple reason that most mental health interventions require no more than an adequately trained mental health human resource. Much emphasis has been placed on the specific role of specialist mental health resources, i.e. psychiatrists, clinical psychologists, psychiatric nurses and psychiatric social workers. The enormous shortage of these mental health specialists, their iniquitous distribution within and between countries and the inefficient way in which they dispense their time, are related to all of the five barriers noted in Panel 1. The *Lancet* series has comprehensively documented the scarcity, inequity and inefficiency of mental health specialists (Saxena *et al.* 2007). Scarcity, an indicator of the absolute number of resources, is a characteristic of all low-income and lower middle-income countries. Low-income countries have 200-fold fewer psychiatrists and psychiatric nurses than high-income countries; the equivalent gaps for clinical psychologists and psychiatric social workers is over 350-fold. This scarcity is unlikely to be significantly ameliorated by increased training as the numbers of specialists being trained each year is so small, and a substantial proportion of these are lost to the low-income world owing to migration to richer countries.

The maldistribution of specialist resources, such that the vast majority work in a few urban areas and an increasing proportion in the private sector, means that the scarcity is even greater for the majority of populations in many countries, i.e. rural or poor people. The final nail in the coffin, and the primary target of the argument for redefining the professional role of specialists, is the inefficiency in how these specialists spend their time. In spite of the vast differences in health systems between high- and low-income countries – which, apart from absolute numbers of human resources, also include the lack of multidisciplinary teams or community mental health systems, weak public health infrastructures and weak social welfare nets – mental health specialists in low-income countries behave in pretty much the same way as their counterparts in high-income countries. In short, they spend most or all of their time in face-to-face clinical work, hospital management and medical student or specialist training.

As I have argued elsewhere (Patel 2009), if all the psychiatrists in India did nothing but see patients every day, limiting their contact to 60 minutes per patient each year, they would altogether see barely 10% of those with serious mental disorders in a year. Unsurprisingly, this figure is consonant with that reported from population-based surveys, which report a treatment gap of 90%. If anything, the situation would be even worse in most other low-income countries. Business as usual will, quite simply, not close the treatment gap for the foreseeable future. A radical revision in our idea of the professional role of specialist mental health human resources is needed.

Rethinking the professional role of mental health specialists

The central role of mental health specialists should shift from striving to ensure the highest standards of individual clinical care to striving to ensure that all those in the populations they serve who need at least basic mental healthcare receive it according to the principles of scientific evidence and protection of their dignity and human rights. Such care must be provided with the philosophy of primary healthcare, and it should have the following attributes: acceptable to the community; affordable; accountable, equitable; and effective, addressing the physical and mental health and social welfare needs of the person affected. This is a tall order indeed, but it is an aspiration, one which is an ultimate goal that the mental health professions should value and affirm, and take steps, however small and incremental, to achieve. I suggest at least four major roles for the mental health professional of the future: supporting community and primary mental healthcare programmes; carrying out essential research, including monitoring and evaluation; building capacity in mental health stakeholders, including their own capacity in public health skills; and advocacy to counter discrimination and protect the human rights of people with mental disorders. I will briefly consider the scope of each of these four roles.

Supporting mental healthcare programmes

The most exciting evidence emerging from low-resource settings in recent years has been the demonstration that mental health treatments can be effectively delivered by lay health workers or community health workers (Patel and Kirkwood 2008). Such evidence in support of task-shifting in mental healthcare is now available for depression, schizophrenia and dementia (see Bolton *et al.* 2003, Chatterjee *et al.* 2003, Dias *et al.* 2008, Rahman *et al.* 2008 for some examples); it is quite likely that as more trials are carried out for other mental disorders, similar evidence will emerge in the future. An integrated population-based mental healthcare plan, based on the principles of task-shifting, has been designed for implementation in India (Patel *et al.* 2009). Such a plan envisages the role of the mental health specialist as the programme leader of the district or population mental health programme. The specialist takes overall responsibility for all clinical aspects of the programme. In principle, this would go much beyond the traditional model of designing and being involved with the training of the community health workers, and would extend to implementing the collaborative model of care that emphasizes continuing support and supervision of the community- or primary care-based workers. Such support and supervision would include regular structured meetings (e.g. where cases are discussed or seen jointly, where personal issues and problems are discussed, etc.). There is ample evidence showing that training alone is not effective (Hodges *et al.* 2001), while in contrast collaborative care models are (for example, see Bower *et al.* 2006 for a systematic review of collaborative care interventions for depression). Such integrated models of care are now being implemented in many populations, often pioneered by non-governmental organizations (NGOs) but increasingly being adopted as models for national mental health programmes as well.

Carrying out priority research

Although there is a growing body of evidence which strengthens the knowledge base to guide mental health programmes, there is also a large evidence gap which needs to be filled. The *Lancet* series on global mental health carried out a systematic priority-setting exercise for research (Tomlinson *et al.*, in press). Priority setting was carried out separately for four groups of disorders: psychoses; depressive and anxiety disorders; substance abuse disorders; and child and adolescent mental disorders. In all four categories, similar research themes emerged as priorities. These priorities could be grouped in three broad domains: health policy and systems research; where and how to deliver existing cost-effective interventions in a low-resource context; and epidemiological research on the broad categories of child and adolescent mental disorders or those pertaining to alcohol and drug abuse, conditions for which even basic descriptive data are lacking from most countries. Mental health specialists must be actively involved as leaders in carrying out this research, which is urgently needed to guide policies and programmes seeking to close the treatment gap. In doing so, collaboration with research disciplines is essential; it is unlikely, or even unnecessary, for clinicians to acquire all the requisite skills to carry out quality research which will have an impact. Collaborations are a critical tool to ensure that scarce human resources are used efficiently by bridging professional communities who have traditionally worked in silos but share a common goal of improving health. However, mental health specialists must all have sufficient research skills to be able to critically assess and evaluate the evidence which is presented to them, to make sense of the extent to which findings may apply to their programmes. Another critical skill, and highly relevant to the role of supporting community and primary care mental health programmes, is that of monitoring and evaluating programmes. At its most basic level, this essentially comprises a clinical audit. At a more sophisticated level, where the objective goes beyond ensuring the quality and accountability of a programme to generating findings which may be generalizable to other programmes, formal research evaluation methodologies may be required.

Building capacity

Capacity to carry out the many diverse tasks needed to close the treatment gap is needed in a diverse range of stakeholders concerned with mental health. Mental health specialists must obviously be actively engaged in building the capacity of front-line health workers, according to the model of task-shifting proposed earlier, to deliver evidence-based care for people with mental disorders. Both training and continuing support and supervision are essential components of such capacity building. One of the greatest barriers for scaling up is the weakness of the user movement in advocating for the needs of persons living with mental disorders. A key role for specialists may be to support users to become more effective advocates, e.g. through networking families, facilitating the establishment of self-help groups (a powerful medium not only for advocacy but also for social support and economic empowerment), and providing appropriate technical support and information. Health policy-makers need to have the capacity to understand how to plan, organize, finance, evaluate and legislate appropriately in mental health; the World Health Organization has prepared a comprehensive set of materials related to building capacity in mental health policy (World Health Organization 2010). Finally, by far the most important group of persons who need capacity building are mental health specialists themselves: as discussed in the final section of this paper, they need training in the diverse public health skills essential to their new roles as leaders in the process of scaling up services.

Advocacy

The common experiences of discrimination described by people with serious mental disorders and the grave levels of human rights abuses have been extensively documented through narratives, research and photojournals (Thornicroft 2006, Thornicroft *et al.* 2009, Patel *et al.*, in press). Quite simply, people with mental disorders are routinely discriminated in every walk of life, and even their basic entitlements (e.g. to health, education and livelihoods) are not addressed uniformly. Advocacy with a diverse range of groups, including the larger community, is an essential strategy to combat discrimination and strengthen institutional mechanisms to protect rights. One of the major barriers to effective advocacy is that the severe mental disorders which are typically associated with the most extreme abuses are precisely those which impair the ability of persons to articulate their grievances and needs effectively, and which lead to people being marginalized and excluded by their own fellow community members. Building capacity to be effective advocates, as mentioned earlier, is a key role of the mental health specialist. The second, and potentially much graver, obstacle is the collusion of the psychiatric and other specialist mental health professional groups with the silence of the global health community. A critical forum for advocacy is within mental health professional societies and groups to make discrimination and human rights a central theme of global psychiatry; until such abuses are addressed comprehensively, the stigma against people with mental disorders – and, indeed, against the mental health professions themselves – will not be eradicated.

Implications for professionalism in low-resource settings

If the mental health professionals are to play a leading role in achieving the ambitious goal of closing the treatment gap, then I have argued that this will require no less than a complete and radical revision of what we do in our day-to-day work. In a nutshell, this would require us to revise our view of ourselves from being primarily clinicians to being primarily clinical public health practitioners. For this to happen, two key elements are needed. First, training programmes for specialists would need to provide a balance between their current emphasis on individual clinical care and the essential skills needed to be an effective public health practitioner. Second, the job profiles of mental health specialists would need to effectively ring-fence time and incentivize performances which directly reflect activities aimed at closing the treatment gaps. I will consider each of these in turn.

Training of mental health specialists

Clinical training in most parts of the world is increasing, emphasizing the need to balance individual biomedical focus with a broader understanding of public health. This is evident in both undergraduate and specialist training schemes. This trend is to be welcomed and indeed strengthened, especially in low-resource settings. Training in public health principles, pedagogical and supervisory skills, basic epidemiology and health service organization and evaluation must be mandatory for all clinical specialists. Many of these can be acquired through formal public health degree training programmes, which are now available as part-time or distance-based learning courses, so that these can be completed concurrently with clinical training. Some skills may need specialized stand-alone courses, in particular for those who have already completed their clinical training. There are several examples of such specialized programmes, ranging from short courses (e.g. Sangath) to formal degree programmes (e.g. Universidade Nova de Lisboa).

Job profiles of mental health specialists

In keeping with the broader set of skills and proficiencies of the new mental health specialist, job profiles must ring-fence time for these roles. I would not wish to prescribe what proportion of time this should be, but at the very least no less than 50% of time should be devoted to the public health agenda of scaling up services, e.g. through community engagement and research. Incentives and rewards based on the achievement of measurable goals according to a range of indicators, such as those proposed by the *Lancet* series on global mental health (Lancet Global Mental Health Group 2007), may be considered as motivators for these new roles. Professional societies must advocate strongly with employers to ensure that such roles are valued and protected in job profiles.

Conclusions

As I have argued elsewhere,

in achieving these public health goals, the role of psychiatrists (and other mental health specialists) will need radical rethinking: put simply, aping the models used in comparatively very well-resourced settings with their veritable armies of diverse mental health professionals (which, ironically, never seem enough to meet the needs of these countries) will not even dent the huge treatment gap in low and middle income countries. (Patel 2009)

Professionalism in psychiatry in resource-poor settings is much more than being a good clinician. Excellence in individual clinical care may be rewarding for the practitioner and the lucky individual who has been able to access this care; however, it has very limited significance from a social justice and equity perspective when the vast majority of others in the same community are denied care. Even those who can access clinical care will not benefit fully, as clinical care alone plays only a limited role in enabling people with mental disorders to lead free, fulfilling and productive lives. It is clear that mental health specialists will need to radically revise their view of themselves and, in so doing, their professional skills and roles, to make a genuine contribution to improving the lives of people with mental disorders and the mental health of the communities they serve.

References

Asuni T (1991). Development of psychiatry in Africa. In S O Okpaku (ed.) *Mental Health in Africa and the Americas Today*. Nashville: Chrisolith Books.

Bolton P, Bass J, Neugebauer R, *et al.* (2003). Group interpersonal psychotherapy for depression in rural Uganda. *Journal of the American Medical Association* **289**, 3117–3124.

Bower P, Gilbody S, Richards D, Fletcher J, Sutton A (2006). Collaborative care for depression in primary care: making sense of a complex intervention. Systematic review and meta-regression. *British Journal of Psychiatry* **189**, 484–493.

Chatterjee S, Patel V, Chatterjee A, Weiss H (2003). Evaluation of a community based rehabilitation model for chronic schizophrenia in a rural region of India. *British Journal of Psychiatry* **182**, 57–62.

Dias A, Dewey M E, D'Souza J, *et al.* (2008). The effectiveness of a home care program for supporting caregivers of persons with dementia in developing countries: a randomised controlled trial from Goa, India. *PloS one* **3**, e2333.

Editorial (2008). A movement for global mental health is launched. *Lancet* **372**, 1274.

Hodges B, Inch C, Silver I (2001). Improving the psychiatric knowledge, skills, and attitudes of primary care physicians, 1995–2000: a review. *American Journal of Psychiatry* **158**, 1579–1586.

Lancet Global Mental Health Group (2007). Scaling up services for mental disorders-a call for action. *Lancet* **370**, 1241–1252.

Patel V (2009). The future of psychiatry in low and middle income countries. *Psychological Medicine* **39**, 1759–1762.

Patel V, Goel D, Desai R (2009). Scaling up services for mental and neurological disorders. *International Health* **1**, 37–44.

Patel V, Kirkwood B (2008). Perinatal depression treated by community health workers. *Lancet* **372**, 868–869.

Patel V, Kleinman A, Saraceno B (in press). Protecting the human rights of people with mental disorders: a call to action for global mental health. In M Dudley, D Silove, F Gale (eds.) *Mental Health & Human Rights*. Oxford: Oxford University Press.

Rahman A, Malik A, Sikander S, Roberts C, Creed F (2008). Cognitive behaviour therapy-based intervention by community health workers for mothers with depression and their infants in rural Pakistan: a cluster-randomised controlled trial. *Lancet* **372**, 902–909.

Sangath (2010). *Leadership in Mental Health* course. http://sangath.com/hm-TrngProgms. html. Last accessed 27 April 2010.

Saraceno B, Van Ommeren M, Batniji R, *et al.* (2007). Barriers to improvement of mental health services in low-income and middle-income countries. *Lancet* **370**, 1164–1174.

Saxena S, Thornicroft G, Knapp M, Whiteford H (2007). Resources for mental health: scarcity, inequity, and inefficiency. *Lancet* **370**, 878–889.

Thornicroft G (2006). *Shunned*. Oxford: Oxford University Press.

Thornicroft G, Brohan E, Rose D, Sartorius N, Leese M (2009). Global pattern of experienced and anticipated discrimination against people with schizophrenia: a cross-sectional survey. *Lancet* **373**, 408–415.

Tomlinson M, Rudan I, Saxena S, Swartz L, Tsai A, Patel V (in press). Setting investment priorities for research in global mental health. *Bulletin of the World Health Organization*.

Universidade Nova de Lisboa (2010). *International Masters in Mental Health Policy and Services* course. www.fcm.unl.pt/gepg/index.php?option= com_content&task=view&id=400& Itemid=420). Last accessed 27 April 2010.

World Health Organization (2010). *Mental Health Policy and Service Guidance* package. www.who.int/mental_health/policy/ essentialpackage1/en/index.html. Last accessed 27 April 2010.

Chapter 7

Professionalism
Australian perspectives

Katinka Morton, Robert Adler and Bruce Singh

Editors' introduction

Professionalism is the responsibility of the profession, who must own it. Society demands that its healthcare providers are of the highest standard and are also knowledgeable and fully skilled. Professionalism is at the core of what psychiatrists do. Playing different clinical and non-clinical roles in different settings to the highest possible standards, the profession also has a major responsibility to ensure that its members behave according to the standards set by the profession.

Using historical accounts from Australia, Morton *et al.* draw parallels with international standards of professionalism and illustrate specific issues in the context of scandals in the 1960s and 1970s. They also raise the issues of intimacy in the context of psychotherapy and the impact of the most intimate thoughts and feelings, making the patient vulnerable and the psychiatrist even more powerful. This power imbalance then leads to debilitating effects associated with control and ambivalent feelings towards therapy and risks, stigmatizing the profession and the patient. Underpinning this is professional self-regulation and the reporting of misconduct. Trust between the patient and the doctor is at the core of any psychotherapeutic relationship. Morton *et al.* point out that professionalism in psychiatry must start at the stage of selection into medical schools. Education within undergraduate medical training and postgraduate psychiatry training, along with lifelong learning related to medical professionalism, is crucial. Expectations of professional standards, values, attitudes and skills by both the public and society on the one hand and the profession itself on the other have to be at the heart of clinical practice in psychiatry.

The Australian context

The evil that men do lives after them,
The good is oft interred with their bones;
Shakespeare, *Julius Caesar*, Act 3, Sc 2

While the focus of this chapter is on professionalism in psychiatry, it is important to recall that unprofessional conduct by psychiatrists taints us all and undermines the trust that our patients have in us as individual psychiatrists as well as in the discipline of psychiatry and medicine in general.

The Australian approach to professionalism is based on international standards of professional conduct in medicine and psychiatry. However, Australian psychiatry has been

Professionalism in Mental Healthcare: Experts, Expertise and Expectations, ed. Dinesh Bhugra and Amit Malik. Published by Cambridge University Press. © Cambridge University Press 2011.

uniquely influenced by instances of unacceptable care, in which patients received care that was neither medically competent nor professional. These incidents have often been highly publicized in the media. The interaction between these incidents, their investigation and the subsequent response of the Australian community has played an important part in establishing clearer expectations of professional conduct in Australian psychiatry.

Australians seeking healthcare currently do so through public or private healthcare systems. The universal public healthcare system, known as Medicare, is funded by public taxes – including a means-tested levy – and includes most inpatient psychiatry in the public sector. Medicare also funds part of the outpatient care of the mentally ill. Private inpatient psychiatric treatment is available to those with private health insurance and those who can afford to pay. Complaints about the public system in psychiatry tend to focus on issues relating to involuntary hospitalization and treatment as well as standards of care provided to public patients.

Australians have historically demonstrated some indifference towards those institutionalized with mental illness (Ash *et al.* 2007), and in this context there have been a number of instances of institutional exploitation of mentally ill patients. A New South Wales psychiatric hospital, Callan Park, was investigated in a Royal Commission in 1960–1961, after the medical superintendent, Dr H R Bailey, went to the media with concerns about neglect of, and cruelty towards, patients. The Inquiry (New South Wales Government 1961) determined that, although some of Dr Bailey's concerns were substantiated, others were 'largely unfounded.' Nonetheless, the report documented 'instances of cruelty to patients', 'evidence of neglect of patients', and 'a small number of male staff … guilty of cruelty.' Recommendations included improvement in the physical circumstances and care of patients, as well as an increased focus on rehabilitation with a view to discharging patients. The unprofessional conduct of staff was directly linked to unacceptable standards of patient care.

The same Dr Bailey was a psychiatrist at Chelmsford Private Hospital, where from 1963 to 1979 he used various combinations of deep sedation, known as deep sleep therapy, often in conjunction with electroconvulsive therapy. Dr Bailey was also engaged in sexual relationships with several of his female patients (Ellard 1991). In the mid 1970s, nursing staff at Chelmsford became increasingly concerned about the medical complications of deep sedation, and the use of 'deep sleep treatment' ended in 1979 after Dr Bailey's exit from Chelmsford.

A Royal Commission was announced in 1988, after a public affairs television programme examined the use of deep sedation at Chelmsford. The fifteen-volume Royal Commission report documented 24 patient deaths, as well as concerns about the physical care of patients, the lack of informed consent and the use of restraint. How the practices at Chelmsford could have continued as long as they did has had direct implications for the structures put in place to ensure that there would be no repeat. It has since been noted that 'the substantial blame was attributed to those who had the power to regulate and control medical practice' (Ellard 1991).

There were also incidents in other Australian states involving serious concerns about patient care. For example, in Queensland there was a Commission of Inquiry into the psychiatric ward at Townsville General Hospital. The Australian community progressively responded to unregulated institutional care with demands for greater regulation, with monitoring and vigilance on behalf of the vulnerable. Progressive deinstitutionalization and increased regulation have had protective effects for the severely mentally ill. Regulatory bodies, including the Royal Australian and New Zealand College of Psychiatrists (RANZCP), medical registration boards and mental health review boards continue to struggle with the challenge of ensuring that mentally ill persons, who are often vulnerable to exploitation by the very nature of their illness, receive the same high standard of care that should be available to all members of the community.

Recently, an Australian doctor, Dr Graham Reeves, became known as 'The Butcher of Bega' in the popular media. Although he worked outside the field of psychiatry, complaints about his professional conduct have had far-reaching consequences for all Australian medical practitioners. The New South Wales Minister for Health announced 'the strongest legislation in the country to protect patients against misconduct by doctors' in May 2008. This legislation included the introduction of 'mandatory reporting by medical practitioners of their colleagues in instances of serious misconduct.' New South Wales is the first Australian state or territory to introduce mandatory reporting, and the link between this and the case of Dr Reeves was made overt by Minister Meagher's statement that 'These stronger laws follow revelations about the handling of complaints about the conduct of Dr Graeme Reeves by regulatory and disciplinary authorities' (Meagher 2008).

As can be seen, legislation has been developed in response to highly publicized cases of unacceptable patient care, whether perpetrated by individual clinicians or within institutional settings. Expectations of professional conduct in Australian psychiatry have undoubtedly been influenced by these cases, but they are also derived from an understanding of the essential features of the psychiatrist–patient relationship and the ethical issues which result.

Professionalism and psychiatry

He was meddling too much in my private life.
Quote attributed to Tennessee Williams,
explaining why he stopped seeing his psychoanalyst

Professionalism, psychiatry and intimacy

In the quote above, Tennessee Williams, explaining why he had stopped seeing his psychoanalyst, refers to his analyst's involvement in his 'private life'. The management of mental illness requires extraordinary intimacy between patient and psychiatrist. A patient's mental illness may impact on every aspect of his or her internal and external world. The treatment of such illness cannot proceed optimally without the psychiatrist understanding not only the patient's symptoms, but also the meaning of these symptoms in the patient's life and internal world. The patient describes the impact of illness on their relationships, employment and finances as well as their experience of themselves and the powerful emotions they experience.

Psychotherapy, particularly intensive psychoanalytic psychotherapy, is associated with greater levels of intimacy than any other treatment because of its nature and duration. In psychodynamic psychotherapies, the exploration of the patient's world is less about their experience of symptoms and response to treatment than it is the treatment itself. The patient and psychiatrist engage in psychotherapy with the expectation that there will be changes to the patient's very self, therefore the patient is expected to entrust the therapist with their most intimate thoughts and feelings, making them potentially vulnerable to exploitation by an unethical therapist who chooses to ignore or even misuse the transference inherent in the relationship.

Although intimacy may be established in a single doctor–patient encounter, the likelihood of intimacy is increased in longer-term therapeutic relationships. Psychiatrists are frequently involved in the long-term care of patients, and the very nature of psychotherapy is such that it involves the disclosure of intimate thoughts and feelings in a way that is much more personal than exposing one's body to various physical treatments in the more physical specialties. These longer-term relationships, and the greater intimacy that results, have been associated with unprofessional conduct such as professional sexual misconduct (PSM). This highly personal disclosure is peculiar to psychiatry and, to a lesser extent, to general practice, which may be the principal explanation for the over-representation of these two areas of medicine in reports of sexual misconduct. It is this intimacy and the resultant power imbalance, combined with the inherent vulnerability of the patient population in psychiatry, that warrant even higher standards of professionalism among psychiatrists.

Professionalism, psychiatry and power imbalances

The unequal disclosure of information, and the patient's reliance on the doctor for medical treatment, results in a power imbalance inherent in all doctor–patient relationships. In psychiatry, this is exaggerated by the debilitating effects of and the stigma associated with mental illness, as well as the power associated with the access that psychiatrists have to Mental Health Acts to enforce treatments and/or hospitalize patients against their will.

This call for an even higher standard of professionalism among psychiatrists is further justified by the consequences of unprofessional behaviour. Quadrio (1992) has explored the consequences of sexual boundary violations on patients receiving psychotherapy. The majority of the 40 women who experienced PSM developed depression, and suicidal ideation was frequent. All experienced a subsequent marked deterioration in interpersonal and occupational functioning, with consequent longer-term disability for most. Also noted were ambivalent feelings towards the abuser, which often compromised subsequent engagement with care and rehabilitation. The combination of deliberate self-harm ideation and difficulties engaging in further treatment is an alarming one, and it further emphasizes the potentially harmful consequences of PSM.

Planning for professionalism in Australian psychiatry

Prominent cases of professional misconduct, and an understanding of the implications of this within the psychiatrist–patient relationship, emphasize the need for very high standards of professionalism within psychiatry. Translating these standards into clinical practice can be considered in terms of:

1. Establishing standards of professional conduct
2. Promoting professional conduct, and
3. Regulating professional conduct.

Standards of professional conduct

While standards of professional conduct in Australia have inevitably been influenced by local events, an approach to professionalism based on extreme examples of unprofessional conduct would be inadequate for a number of reasons. First, some professional misconduct has been noted to be somewhat recalcitrant towards increasingly explicit professional codes of conduct for psychiatrists, with persisting complaints of PSM despite these codes (Kiel 2006).

Second, patients are often reluctant to report or delay reporting professional misconduct. They may be unsure of the limits of acceptable behaviour, influenced by the power imbalance inherent in the doctor–patient relationship; their illness may prohibit engagement in the complaints process; and many are simply embarrassed to admit that they 'voluntarily' engaged in a sexual relationship with their psychiatrist, believing him or her to be in love with them. Perhaps most worryingly, patients may not complain because they believe that there will not be any response to their concerns, that cronyism still persists in the medical profession. For all these reasons, reports of professional misconduct are likely to underestimate the true community prevalence and be biased towards the more extreme examples.

Finally, it is only a very small proportion of doctors who are involved in serious professional misconduct. Standards of professional conduct should be relevant to all medical practitioners and should therefore aim to improve professional conduct, rather than only delineate misconduct.

Standards of professional conduct are not limited to formal guidelines. A number of Australian psychiatrist authors and teachers have produced descriptions of professional conduct that have become standards in themselves. Australian psychiatrist John Ellard encouraged psychiatrists to imagine that one wall of their consulting room is transparent, with a 'grandstand of (my) senior colleagues' watching their clinical conduct (Ellard 1998). In considering whether their professional boundaries are appropriate, the self-regulating psychiatrist is encouraged to consider 'the judgement (of their peers)'. This simple exercise, and the resultant standard of 'being able to defend one's clinical behaviour to a group of colleagues', has become an implicit expectation of professional conduct in Australian psychiatry.

Other Australian psychiatrists have made similar comments that serve to guide clinical practice, such as 'a psychiatrist should be friendly towards patients, yet not try to be their friend' (B. Singh, personal communication, 2005), and 'it is always the patient's prerogative to behave badly' (Quadrio (1992), when emphasizing that the psychiatrist, not the patient, is responsible for any boundary violations). Such observations have influenced and guided Australian clinicians and have contributed to Australian approaches to professionalism.

Australia has not been without more formal standards of professional conduct, however, as demanded by failures in self-regulation. These standards are most obviously imposed and regulated by state medical registration boards. The challenges facing these boards are not peculiar to Australia. In recent years in the UK there have been a number of well-known cases that have raised questions about the effectiveness of self-regulation of the medical profession. The case of Harold Shipman, possibly the most serious serial killer in the UK, and the tragic deaths of children undergoing cardiac surgery in Bristol led to questions about the effectiveness of the General Medical Council (GMC). One response has been the inclusion of community or non-medical members on medical boards in Australia and on the GMC in the UK. The GMC also developed a code of conduct for medical practitioners, *Good Medical Practice*, which 'sets out the principles and values on which good practice is founded; these principles together describe medical professionalism in action' (General Medical Council 2006).

Good Medical Practice has been adapted to the Australian context by a number of state and territory medical boards. Currently, it is undergoing revision through an extensive consultation process to make it a nationally agreed document in anticipation of the introduction of national registration and accreditation in July 2010. *Good Medical Practice* is increasingly being used by medical boards as the benchmark against which to measure the standards of ethical and professional conduct of all doctors registered to practise medicine in Australia, as well as setting out the principles that should characterize good medical practice.

In addition to the traditional ethical pillars of respect, beneficence, non-maleficence and justice, the draft national Good Medical Practice emphasizes the central role of **trust** in the doctor–patient relationship; the importance of making the care of one's patients one's first concern and recognizing that each patient is unique; that integrity, truthfulness, dependability and compassion are key attributes of the good doctor; that 'good communication underpins every aspect of good medical practice.' The draft code states

Professionalism embodies all the qualities described (in the preceding paragraphs), and includes self-awareness and self-reflection. Doctors are expected to reflect regularly on whether they are practising effectively, what is happening in their relationship with patients and colleagues, and on their own health and well-being. They keep their skills and knowledge up to date, refine and develop their clinical judgment as they gain experience, and contribute to their profession.

The code addresses matters relating to clinical care, working with other health professionals in the healthcare system in Australia, professional behaviour, the importance of maintaining one's own health, and teaching and research. The code is of necessity very general, as it is intended to outline principles applicable to all areas of medical practice. It is therefore not specific to psychiatry.

Promoting professionalism in Australian psychiatry

The introduction to professionalism in psychiatry should commence before subspecialty training. The challenge is to understand how good professional conduct can be promoted and unprofessional conduct prevented. It is increasingly clear that even the best education, regulations and legislation do not guarantee professional conduct. In particular, educating the community about the reasonable expectations they may have of their medical practitioner, through guidelines such as Good Medical Practice, must proceed with the awareness that contradictory information may abound within popular culture, most notably in the media.

Selection to medical school

Australia is currently experiencing significant medical workforce shortages. As a result, a significant proportion of Australia's doctors are International Medical Graduates who completed their medical school training before coming to Australia. They are drawn from many different ethnic, cultural and religious groups whose understanding of community expectations may differ markedly from those of Australian graduates. Over the next 5 years the number of Australian medical graduates will increase markedly, and these doctors will be eligible to apply for the RANZCP specialty training following completion of a 12-month internship. Selection to medical school is therefore a key opportunity to select future Australian psychiatrists.

Medical schools have historically utilized academic criteria for the selection of medical students. Increasingly, however, both the community and medical schools have advocated assessment of some non-cognitive qualities, in addition to academic results, to determine entry into medicine. It has been argued that non-cognitive characteristics, in addition to academic results, may better identify applicants who are more likely to succeed in medical school and become 'good doctors' than the use of academic results alone (Ferguson *et al.* 2002,

Wagoner 2006). In this context, medical schools in Australia have increasingly incorporated some non-cognitive assessments into their intake processes.

There are, however, significant concerns associated with use of non-cognitive criteria in selection for medical school. Their application is significantly more demanding of resources than the historical reliance on academic record alone (Albanese *et al.* 2003, Wagoner 2006). It could be argued that the expense is justified when considered in the context of the costs for the community of both medical education and unprofessional conduct. However, there is a lack of consensus about the reliability and predictive validity of these measures and about which qualities are associated with professionalism, as well as uncertainty about how these qualities are best assessed. Different authors argue for the utility of various forms of interviews and objective, structured clinical examinations (Stern *et al.* 2005, Wagoner 2006) but note the potential for these to be undermined by various factors, including the highly motivated, resourceful applicant (Albanese *et al.* 2003). In the absence of reliable, valid measures, the most alarming concern raised about the use of non-cognitive measures for medical school applicants is the potential for a lack of fairness and a reduction in diversity (Wagoner 2006).

Non-cognitive selection criteria to medical schools, whether behaviour- or values-based, have not been shown to predict subsequent professional behaviour as yet. Medical schools are under pressure to have efficient selection processes that are both rigorous and defensible under appeal. In this context, the Australian Medical Council (AMC), responsible for the accreditation of all Australian medical schools, does not require them to utilize non-cognitive measures (Australian Medical Council 2009). Medical schools within Australia are required to have 'clearly defined selection policy and procedures' that are published and hence publicly available. The AMC stipulates only that these measures should 'minimise discrimination and bias,' and that the 'intended relationship between selection criteria, the objectives of the course, and graduate outcomes is stated.'

Within medical schools

The current evidence suggests that, at present, medical schools cannot be confident of their ability to exclude inappropriate applicants. Indeed, it is unlikely that any medical school selection process will ever be able to offer an absolute guarantee in this regard. Optimizing professional attitudes and skills during medical school, and ensuring that there are appropriate processes in place for the exclusion of medical students about whom unresolvable concerns have been identified, are important in this context.

The AMC (2009) currently requires all Australian medical schools to have 'procedures for identifying and dealing with students with needs related to mental health or professional behaviour issues.' Recently, Parker and Wilkinson (2008) advocated the development of a consistent, specific set of procedures in response to such problems. They noted that interviews during the admission process do not prevent the entry of a small number of students who perform at a satisfactory level academically but who demonstrate 'persistent unprofessional behaviour'. With reference to the UK's GMC (2007) publication, *Medical Students: Professional Behaviour and Fitness to Practise*, the authors argue for a nationally consistent approach implemented within medical schools (rather than by state medical boards). They propose an initial process of data gathering to establish a 'case law collection' of students requiring serious disciplinary action.

For the majority of medical students who do not demonstrate these concerns, there has also been consideration of the training required to promote the theoretical knowledge and attitudes necessary for professional conduct. This training occurs both through formal education programmes, such as that conducted by White (2004) in Tasmania, and also through the apprenticeship model utilized in Australian medical schools. Reports of the sexual harassment of undergraduate medical students are of particular concern in this context, with the potential to promote inappropriate conduct at a crucial stage of attitude formation. Quadrio (1992) appeals for a challenge to sexism within the profession and questions the promotion of 'driving, aggressive, highly masculinised' values within clinicians. Those charged with training medical students must be clear about their influence in terms of both formal teaching and the modelling of professional conduct.

Selection for psychiatry training

Within Australia, the standards for specialty training in psychiatry are set by the RANZCP. Doctors selected to specialize in psychiatry are required to complete a 5-year training programme that includes a number of mandatory training rotations using an apprenticeship model, with accredited supervisors. In addition, there are a number of formal assessments, including written and clinical examinations.

The RANZCP selection process includes a written application, a structured interview, a work performance certificate and the submission of referees' reports. The state and territory Branch Training Committees responsible for selection will consider all these factors in an attempt to ensure that any history of unprofessional behaviour is known and considered. In this way, candidates with a history of past unprofessional behaviour may be considered inappropriate for RANZCP training.

The importance of professional behaviour in specialty training is recognized by the AMC in its accreditation of specialist college standards (AMC 2008). In particular, the declared outcome of all specialist education is stated to be 'to produce medical specialists who have demonstrated the requisite knowledge, skills and professional attributes necessary for independent practice.' The RANZCP certainly recognizes the importance of the selection of suitable candidates and is supported by the AMC in doing so. Research into the validity of these selection measures is limited by the multiple variables, including subsequent training, which influence outcomes for individual trainees.

Teaching within psychiatry training

Once selected to train in psychiatry, registrars are required to demonstrate that they have acquired the knowledge, attitude and skills required by the training curriculum during 3 years of basic training and 2 years of advanced training. The RANZCP curriculum stipulates that 'Trainees share the responsibility of upholding the integrity of the medical profession and should develop an attitude whereby they recognise the privileges accorded to them.' The apprenticeship model is a vital component of this training. All RANZCP supervisors must complete training to be accredited, and professional conduct is emphasized within this training. With an emphasis on the apprenticeship model, trainees work closely with their supervisors and are expected to observe and demonstrate professional conduct in their clinical work throughout training. In turn, the importance of professional conduct is emphasized to trainees, with the inclusion of this conduct as a requirement for the satisfactory completion of training rotations.

The RANZCP is currently undertaking a major review of the curriculum. This review provides another opportunity to improve the training necessary to ensure that the psychiatrists of the future conduct themselves in a professional manner.

Post-Fellowship requirements for continuing medical education

Once training is successfully completed, RANZCP trainees become 'Fellows' of the College. All Fellows are expected to participate in the RANZCP's Continuing Professional Development (CPD) Program. The CPD Program has the declared aim of facilitating the 'participation of Fellows in ongoing professional development activities' and to 'encourage a culture within the College of review and reflection on professional practices.'

Adler and Mathieson (1998) described the progression of continuing education from being 'largely the responsibility of the individual' within the RANZCP Program and mandatory Continuing Medical Education (CME) and recertification as 'a very recent development.' More than 10 years later, his comment about CME becoming mandatory 'insidiously rather than by legislation' remains pertinent. The CPD Program is not currently mandatory for Fellows of the RANZCP, nor is CPD participation a uniform requirement for medical registration across all Australian states and territories. There continue to be major challenges, such as optimizing on line learning and ensuring that the CPD Program is relevant for psychiatrists in all areas of practice.

Ellard (1991) described the formation of the RANZCP's CPD Program and Practice Standards Committee. Despite the Chelmsford Royal Commission, many psychiatrists continued to see 'monitoring as a threat to (their) clinical independence.' Ellard argued that, far from threatening our independence, the purpose of external scrutiny was 'protecting our patients and preserving our reputation.'

The RANZCP has recognized this responsibility with the development of a first Code of Ethics in 1992 and the ongoing development of Position Statements (RANZCP 2005) concerning specific ethical issues within the community. The Code of Ethics (RANZCP 2004) is currently under review and faces the ongoing challenge of representing contemporary values of the community and the profession.

Regulating professional conduct

Promoting professionalism cannot obviate the need for regulation given the very serious consequences of even isolated instances of unprofessional conduct. In Australia, much of this regulation is performed by state and territory medical registration boards established by state legislation. The Coalition of Australian Governments (Federal, State and Territory) are currently developing a framework for national registration and accreditation of ten health professions, including medicine. The movement towards a National Health Registration and Accreditation Act, rather than a national Medical Practice Act, to regulate the medical profession specifically has raised a number of concerns, including the appropriateness of the Act for multiple disciplines. The uniform implementation of a standardized Act will provide new opportunities for the examination and review of the professional conduct of health practitioners across Australia and, hopefully, better protection of the public.

Numerous highly publicized instances of PSM by psychiatrists over the past 20–30 years have led the RANZCP to articulate increasingly clear expectations with regard to the matter of sexual relations between psychiatrists, their patients and former patients. In addition to regulation through the medical boards, Australian psychiatrists are now subject to discipline by the RANZCP, including loss of their College Fellowship.

Quadrio (1992) has argued that increased medical regulation alone cannot address professional misconduct. In particular, Quadrio has argued that the broader social context must be considered to minimize PSM. The community must be confident of the conduct that they may expect of their psychiatrist, and any concerns that they have about this conduct must be addressed. In the same way that the educational environment and experience of future doctors must be considered more broadly than the formal teaching that they receive, the expectations of patients must be considered within the context of their community's gender roles and values.

Conclusions

Expectations of professionalism in the Australian context have been influenced by a number of instances of unprofessional conduct by psychiatrists. These have resulted in important changes in legislation with implications for clinical practice, but perhaps even more important is the damage done to the reputation of psychiatry by such conduct. Australian psychiatry now has far greater professional expectations of itself and promotes professional conduct, rather than simply responding to unprofessional conduct. Although some of the precedents which shaped Australian legislation and expectations may be peculiar to Australia and the Australian system of healthcare, the ongoing challenges of both improving professional conduct and responding to misconduct are similar to those which are faced internationally.

Postscript

From 1 July 2010 the medical profession in Australia was regulated by a single medical board, the Medical Board of Australia, under a single Health Practitioner Regulation National Law enacted in each state and territory. For the first time there is a nationally consistent approach to the registration, accreditation and regulation of the medical profession, along with nine other health professions, throughout Australia.

References

Adler R, Mathieson S (1998). Throwing out the bathwater: preparing psychiatrists for the 21st century. *Australasian Psychiatry* **6**, 296–302.

Albanese M A, Snow M H, Skochelak S E, Huggett K N, Farrell P M (2003). Assessing personal qualities in medical school admissions. *Academic Medicine* **78**, 313–321.

Ash D, Benson A, Dunbar L, *et al.* (2007). Mental health services in Australia. In G Meadows, B Singh, M Grigg (eds.) *Mental Health in Australia: Collaborative Community Practice*. Oxford: Oxford University Press, pp. 63–98.

Australian Medical Council (2008). Amended document, replacing Part B of the Australian Medical Council's guidelines, accreditation of specialist medical education and training and professional development programs: standards and procedures, 2002. In *Assessing Specialist Medical Education and Training*. www.amc.org.au/index.php/accreditation-aamp-recognition-mainmenu-188/specialist-colleges-mainmenu-189. Last accessed 1 April 2009.

Australian Medical Council (2009). Assessment and accreditation of Australian medical schools: standards and procedures, 2009. In *Australian Medical Council Standards and Processes MedSAC*. www.amc.org.au/images/Medschool.standards.pdf. Last accessed 1 April 2009.

Ellard J (1991). Chelmsford and its aftermath. *Psychiatric Bulletin* **15**, 686–688.

Ellard J (1998). Professional boundaries: the forbidden territories. *Modern Medicine of Australia* July, 46–49.

Ferguson E, James D, Madeley L (2002). Factors associated with success in medical school: systematic review of the literature. *BMJ* **324**, 952–957.

General Medical Council (2006). *Good Medical Practice Guidance for Doctors*. www.gmcuk.org/guidance/good_medical_practice/GMC_GMP.pdf. Last accessed 12 May 2009.

General Medical Council (2007). Medical students: professional behaviour and fitness to practice. In *General Medical Council: Regulating Doctors, Ensuring Good Medical Practice*. www.gmcuk.org/education/undergraduate/undergraduate_policy/professional_behaviour.asp. Last accessed 4 March 2009.

Kiel H (2006). Drugs, sex and the risk of recidivism: psychiatry in the witness box. *Psychiatry, Psychology and Law* **13**, 132–142.

Meagher R (New South Wales Minister for Health) (2008). *Landmark Legislation to Deal with Misconduct by Doctors*. Sydney: New South Wales Government Department of Health, 7 May. www.health.nsw.gov.au/news/2008/20080507_01.html. Last accessed 16 April 2010.

New South Wales Government (1961). Royal Commission of Inquiry in respect of certain matters relating to Callan Park Mental Hospital. In *State Records Authority of New South Wales*. http://investigator.records.nsw.gov/Entity.aspx?Path=%5CAgency%5C4960. Last accessed 4 March 2009.

Parker M H, Wilkinson D (2008). Dealing with "rogue" medical students: we need a nationally consistent approach based on "case law". *Medical Journal of Australia* **189**, 626–628.

Quadrio C (1992). Sex and gender and the impaired therapist. *Australian and New Zealand Journal of Psychiatry* **26**, 346–363.

Royal Australian and New Zealand College of Psychiatrists (2004). *The RANZCP Code of Ethics*. www.ranzcp.org/images/stories/ranzcp-attachments/Resources/College_Statements/Code_of_Ethics.pdf. Last accessed 29 April 2010.

Royal Australian and New Zealand College of Psychiatrists (2005). Ethics statement: sexual relationships with patients. In *The Royal Australian and New Zealand College of Psychiatrists Ethical Guidelines*. www.ranzcp.org/images/stories/ranzcp-attachments/Resources/College_Statements/Ethical_Guidelines/eg08.pdf. Last accessed 1 April 2009.

Stern D T, Frohna A Z, Gruppen L D (2005). The prediction of professional behaviour. *Medical Education* **39**, 75–82.

Wagoner N E (2006). Admission to medical school: selecting applicants with the potential for professionalism. In D T Stern (ed.) *Measuring Medical Professionalism*. Oxford: Oxford University Press, pp. 235–263.

White G E (2004). Setting and maintaining professional boundaries: an educational strategy. *Medical Education* **38**, 903–910.

Chapter

8

Can professionalism be taught? Lessons for undergraduate medical education

Robert A. Murden

Editors' introduction

Professionalism can be taught and learnt using a number of different strategies and methods. It is important that professionals learn the fundamentals and the components of professionalism at an early stage. It is desirable that models used to teach professionalism are in the appropriate social and cultural context, taking into account values defined by society. Murden highlights the strategies which can be used to learn about and teach professionalism. From mentoring, role modelling, narrative or through example, different strategies may have different roles. Murden emphasizes that teaching by itself is not enough and needs to be evaluated. Clinicians must also be aware of the reasons and strategies to identify or predict unprofessional behaviours. It is easy to identify these in managed environments. Those who are purely in private practice may be more difficult to identify at an early stage. Any such identification must also have an element of remediation built into the process. Some unprofessional attitudes and behaviours can be identified earlier or even in medical school settings. On the other hand, there is evidence that some aspects of professionalism may decline during medical training. It is possible to identify deficiencies and put remedial action in place. The cost of training a doctor and subsequently a psychiatrist is huge, and it is for the profession to ensure that standards are met and maintained. Murden argues cogently that by changing the environment which dominates the learning of professionalism, it should be possible to achieve sustainable long-term goals. The efforts have to be intensive and longitudinal rather than simply here and now and then forgetting about it. Using multiple models to teach professionalism will enable a sea change in attitudes and beliefs about professionalism.

Introduction

There is currently a great emphasis on professionalism in medical schools and in postgraduate training programmes in the United States and internationally. Sometimes this emphasis is on the evaluation of professionalism, and at other times it is on the teaching of professionalism. Although there seems to be a clear consensus that maximizing professionalism among physicians is desirable, there are broad differences in proposed meanings and definitions of professionalism, in methods to evaluate it and teach it, in the effectiveness of efforts to improve professionalism and in beliefs that professionalism is inherent versus learnt. This chapter will address the question of whether professionalism can be effectively taught, by examining what it means to teach professionalism, proposed strategies to teach it, evidence of

Professionalism in Mental Healthcare: Experts, Expertise and Expectations, ed. Dinesh Bhugra and Amit Malik. Published by Cambridge University Press. © Cambridge University Press 2011.

effectiveness of interventions aimed at teaching or improving professionalism and evidence of ability to identify or predict unprofessional behaviour.

What does it mean to teach professionalism?

Professionalism, and the professionalism that can be taught (which requires an assessment component), may be distinct entities. In one of the primary texts on professionalism education, Hafferty notes that 'Professionalism lies in an interface between possession of specialized knowledge, and using that knowledge for the betterment of others' (Hafferty 2000). Similarly, Smith states that professionalism is progressing from lay person to physician and accepting the physician role in society (Smith 2005). This meaning of professionalism refers to acquiring the mantle of the profession and has traditionally been learnt by example (Coulehan 2005), role model (Steinert *et al.* 2007) and narrative (Coulehan 2005).

Conversely, others have defined professionalism as a set of skills, knowledge, attitudes, values, virtues and behaviours (Rees and Knight 2007), much of which can be measured and expressly taught. Furthermore, within this broad definition there may be a distinction between what is labelled as humanism, a deep-seated conviction about obligations to others, and professionalism, a defined set of professional attitudes and behaviours (Stern *et al.* 2008). These distinctions are important because humanism, which would include elements of morality and values, has been noted to be well formed in most medical students at the start of medical school (Huddle 2005). Thus, there is some debate as to how much students can change these well-formed views, although it has been suggested that schools can inculcate desired values (Swick *et al.* 1999) and that humanism can be promoted by setting expectations, creating experiences and evaluating expected behaviours (Stern *et al.* 2008). It is more apparent that professionalism – defined as a set of behaviours, skills, knowledge and attitudes – is potentially teachable. Multiple strategies to teach this notion of professionalism are explored in the next section.

Learning the professionalism of Hafferty and Smith occurs in the culture of medical school and residency, where examples, narratives and role modelling occur. To improve this learning would require changes in the cultures of medical schools. There is wide acknowledgement that current cultures hold many negative features that detract from the cultural assimilation of the desired form of professionalism. For one, medicine is an increasingly technological profit centre with increased opportunities for physicians to make money from commercial relationships, increased expectation of cure by patients and decreased satisfaction with personal interactions by all parties (Coulehan 2005). Associated financial changes often cause faculty to increase clinical effort at the expense of teaching effort (West and Shanafelt 2007), and that, coupled with the previously mentioned ties to commercial concerns, exacerbates the central paradox in medicine – the tension between altruism and self-interest (Coulehan 2005).

Many people decry the so-called disavowed or hidden curriculum (Ginsburg *et al.* 2003) formed from this culture, which often rewards students and residents for unprofessional behaviour. Medical students complain that they are admonished for the same behaviours they observe in their teachers (Stern and Papadakis 2006, Brainard and Brislen 2007, Leo and Eagen 2008). Rewards for gaming the system, expediency and promoting efficiency may inhibit or undercut the development of good moral reasoning and student attitudes towards professionalism (Hafferty 2000, Brainard and Brislen 2007). Stresses in students, residents and faculty contribute to unprofessional behaviours (West and Shanafelt 2007) and to faculty frequently working in crisis mode, which provides poor role modelling (Brainard and Brislen 2007). The extent of this hidden curriculum was documented in a study in which evaluators followed clinical medical school teachers and recorded the teaching examples utilized. Only 5/182 examples emphasized altruism, confidentiality, non-malfeasance, optimism or self-awareness, whereas 22/182 emphasized scepticism, physician convenience and self-protection, and 52/182 emphasized the hierarchy of medical personnel and an industry of efficiency (Stern 1996). Finally, Hafferty notes that medical school mission statements, which often emphasize the development of professionalism, are frequently poorly aligned with the medical curriculum, which emphasizes the acquisition of technical knowledge (Hafferty 2000). This problematic culture of medical schools must be changed if this type of professionalism is to be learnt/improved.

Proposed strategies to teach professionalism

Suggested proposals for teaching professionalism fall into two categories: specific teaching of sets of knowledge, skills, attitudes and behaviours that can be measured; and more general approaches to globally improve professionalism. The former encompass curricular coursework that has been applied, and often tested, to date. The latter are more theoretical approaches that have been suggested, but generally not applied, or at least not tested for effectiveness.

A 1999 survey of US medical schools found that 89.7% offered some listed instruction in professionalism, including 55.2% that assess behaviours and 33.6% that include faculty development (Swick *et al.* 1999). This instruction ran from a single lecture/course or white coat ceremony to longitudinal integrated courses, mostly in the first 2 years of medical school. Most specific instruction is in areas such as ethics, humanities and doctor–patient relationships (Hafferty 2000). A 2-day meeting of the Gold Humanism Foundation further discovered that teaching humanism is generally divided into specific courses studying the humanities and training students in communication and cultural diversity, and more general approaches of experiential and service learning and reflection (Stern *et al.* 2008). Evidence of the effectiveness of this type of teaching of professionalism is included in the next section.

Much more has been written concerning broad proposals to globally improve professionalism. Most of these focus on improving the culture of medical schools and/or improving the ability of faculty to provide ideal teaching. Coulehan notes that we do a good job of talking the talk (teaching the above areas) but a poor job of walking the walk (providing good role models) because we do not focus on the latter (Coulehan 2005). He advocates developing a large cadre of very professional teachers/role models, increasing self-awareness and narrative competence and increasing community service in order to globally improve professionalism. West and Shanafelt similarly advocate good role models, promoting a culture of caring and promoting physician wellbeing as the best methods to improve professionalism (West and Shanafelt 2007). Leo and Eagen suggest a very student-oriented approach which includes involving students in the curriculum and obtaining student support, evaluating everyone on professionalism (not just students), providing rewards for high professionalism (not just punishment for low ratings) and physician development to reinforce the reasons to teach professionalism (Leo and Eagen 2008). Hafferty suggests that medical schools need to emphasize professionalism much more than technical competence, that the hidden curriculum must be addressed and that service and reflection are important (Hafferty 2000). Shrank, Reed and Jernstedt suggest adding incentives for medical students and faculty to improve professionalism, including having specific and separate professionalism grades for students and education/professionalism relative value units (RVUs) for faculty (Shrank *et al.* 2004). Lastly, Cruess and Cruess suggest eight requirements for adequately improving medical school teaching of professionalism (Cruess and Cruess 2006). One is learning the cognitive base of professionalism. The others are the more global areas of institutional support, experiential learning, role modelling, faculty development, assessment, environmental change and continuity of professional learning. These articles demonstrate consistent themes of reducing faculty stress, improving role models, rewards, reflection, community and other experiences and improving the medical school culture.

Several even more general approaches emphasize the processes that learners need to go through to attain professionalism. For instance, Huddle suggests that the most important task of the teacher of professionalism is not to convey moral abstractions, but to reinforce the moral emotions that sustain moral responsiveness in competing situations (Huddle 2005). The theory of planned behaviours notes that behaviour comes from intention for behaviour, modified by attitudes, perceived norms and ease of carrying out the behaviour (Archer *et al.* 2008) (see Chapter 14 for more details). Aligning norms and ease with desired attitudes would therefore maximize desired behaviours. It has been suggested that we should teach students how to negotiate and balance misaligned norms and attitudes because, when faced with choices between professionalism ideals and behaviours expected by their supervisors which may conflict with these ideals, students tend to make choices that maximize their grades, evaluations and reputations (Ginsburg *et al.* 2003). Similarly, Rees and Knight note that attitudes are poor predictors of social behaviour when external constraints (such as social norms) are strong, and that long-term behaviour in a manner discordant from internal attitudes leads to dissonance that individuals resolve by altering either behaviours or attitudes (Rees and Knight 2007). They suggest having a narrative discussion after discordant behaviours to help student self-awareness, and to alter the hidden curriculum so that social norms do not discourage inherently positive attitudes towards professionalism. Finally, it is suggested that attitude–behaviour consistency is highest when attitudes are obtained experientially, not didactically (Archer *et al.* 2008).

Selected additional strategies include assigning the best role models to trainees who need to improve their professionalism the most (Huddle 2005), understanding that role modelling without reflection may not be sufficient to get the point across (Stern and Papadakis 2006) and understanding that the process of evaluation is educational because students value that which is evaluated (Stern *et al.* 2008). As noted above, many of these suggestions are theoretical, but some have been tried. The next section reviews findings of educational effectiveness.

Effectiveness of interventions to teach/improve professionalism

Unfortunately, despite a great deal of emphasis on professionalism, and nearly all medical schools having some coursework in it, there is little evidence that any specific interventions have made significant improvements (Hafferty 2000). This is particularly true of attempts to improve attitudes. A large review of studies assessing attitudes towards professionalism and whether they change found that most studies focused on attitudes towards individual attributes such as ethics, doctor–patient relationships and cultural competency (Jha *et al.* 2007). Assessments utilized were scales, vignettes and questionnaires. No intervention showed significant attitude changes over time. This is consistent with prior studies showing a lack of ability to change attitudes in areas such as aging (Murden *et al.* 1986), and with previously noted beliefs that attitudes are often well formed in incoming medical students and are thus hard to change.

Individual courses designed to improve skills have, on the other hand, shown modest benefits. One study examined 960 students who participated in small group discussions designed to improve moral reasoning skills. Those students who took more than 20 hours of coursework significantly improved moral reasoning skills after the coursework, whereas those who took less than 20 hours had no significant pre- to post-course improvement (Self *et al.* 1998). Modest benefits of improved self-reported empathy and humanism were reported when the Harvard curriculum changed to a problem-based learning style with emphasis in those areas (Moore *et al.* 1994). A significant improvement from 63 to 70% preferred responses to ethics vignettes was reported following a 58-hour ethics course over 2 years (Goldie *et al.* 2002). A short course (1.5 hours of vignette discussion) on general professionalism skills showed improvement from 17 to 38% excellent scores before to 24 to 76% after on professionalism vignettes (Boenink *et al.* 2005). A recent study of urology residents and faculty showed that a series of lectures on evaluating professionalism led to score increases from a mean of six to a mean of eight on a nine-point scale on demonstrating respect, showing commitment to ethical principles and being sensitive to culture (Joyner and Vemulakonda 2007). Thus, disparate studies have shown that individual courses designed to improve specific professionalism skill sets can show improvement in those skill sets. One caveat to this finding is understanding the role of the assessment of professionalism. This can be problematic, as one study showed that multiple evaluators of an Objective Structured Clinical Exam in professionalism often differed markedly in their evaluations of the students, even in some instances agreeing on the observed behaviour but labelling it both very professional and very unprofessional (Mazor *et al.* 2007). A discussion of assessment of professionalism is beyond the scope of this chapter but is important in knowing whether or not we have taught professionalism successfully.

Evidence of ability to identify or predict unprofessional behaviour

In addition to efforts to teach professionalism to all students, many schools have programmes specifically to identify, presumably for the purposes of remediation, students with unprofessional behaviours. Sometimes this consists of professionalism portfolios for all students. More commonly it consists of systems of reporting unprofessional actions. One described system mandates reports of worrisome behaviour to clerkship/course directors (Papadakis *et al.* 2001). The directors review them and, if felt to be serious, they are placed in the student's permanent file. Most reports were noted in the first 2 years of medical school. Areas for evaluation included unmet professional responsibilities, lack of effort, diminished relationships with patients and families and diminished relationships with the healthcare team. Due to the more serious nature of actions in the clinical clerkships, if two or more reports were received in clinical clerkships, or two or more in preclinical courses plus one in a clinical clerkship, this was included in the Dean's evaluation letter for residency application. A total of 3% of students were cited during their 4 years of medical school within the duration of this study.

One school started a programme to encourage identification of professionalism problems for the purposes of remediation by establishing Early Concern Notes (Ainsworth and Szauter 2006). These can be submitted by any faculty, and faculty are encouraged to use a low threshold for submission. They are not retained in the student's permanent file, and remediation efforts are undertaken when concern notes are submitted. Remediation results and percentage of students identified were not reported,

A similar programme allows any teacher/preceptor to submit forms describing professionalism incidents in the areas of relationships, responsibility, respect for patients, honesty, integrity, communication skills, critique, maturity and mood disorders or chemical dependency (Phelan *et al.* 1993). If two or more forms are submitted, an identified student meets with the department chair or the academic progress committee and the assistant dean for student affairs. Over the course of time reported in this paper, 6% of students had at least one form submitted, and 2% had at least two. Remediation efforts were not reported.

Another similar study from Australia reported referring students to a personal and professional development committee if they had problems in the areas of responsibility/reliability, honesty/integrity, doctor–patient relationships, compassion, respect, relating to others, discrimination, participation and self-appraisal (Parker *et al.* 2008). Students were referred to the committee if a professor discovered an issue that he or she could not resolve. Over the length of this study, 19% of students were referred to this committee; however, after committee review only about a quarter of those, or 5.5% of all students during the time period of the study, were interviewed by the committee. Most problems were in the areas of participation or reliability.

Another school reported a pyramid of actions for reported unprofessional behaviour (Hickson *et al.* 2007). Single incidents are managed by informal conversations, non-punitive interventions are used for patterns, action plans are implemented when interventions failed and disciplinary action is taken when plans failed. Only 3% of students received more than one complaint. Of all complaintees, 60% improve, and 20% leave the institution or fail to graduate.

This identification has also been reported on an individual clerkship basis. A survey of US psychiatry clerkship directors showed that 96% evaluate professionalism, 18% with a separate form and 82% as part of the overall clerkship evaluation (Bennett *et al.* 2005). The primary goals of evaluation were to identify problem behaviours (87%), provide feedback (84%), support grades (64%) or identify exemplary behaviour (51%). Remediation for identified problem behaviour included mentorship, repeating the clerkship and referral for mental health treatment. Success of remediation was not reported. This study revealed that 6% of reporting schools identified four or more students a year with problems, and 70% identified one to three students per year.

These reported systems show that the identification of students with professionalism problems is possible. Interestingly, a remarkably similar 2 to 6% of students were identified by each of the different systems, suggesting that this might be the expected number of students with problems, and that all reported systems might be equally effective at identifying students with problem behaviours. Other than the report of 60% of identified students improving at Vanderbilt, however (Hickson *et al.* 2007), results of remediation efforts have not been reported. Thus, it is not clear to what extent we can improve, or teach, professionalism to students with identified unprofessional behaviours.

Several studies have examined predictor variables for unprofessional behaviour. One looked at data starting with admissions variables and continuing through standardized patient ratings in the Med 2 year, and correlated those with subsequent clerkship professionalism scores and appearances at the academic review board. The only three variables which correlated were decreased compliance with obtaining required immunizations, decreased compliance with completing required course evaluations and increased self-assessment of ability compared with evaluators' assessments (Stern *et al.* 2005).

Another study looked at students identified with professionalism deficiencies in the areas of poor process skills, paternalism, extreme shyness/poor communication and negative attitudes towards the course, during a first-semester, year-1 doctor–patient relationship and interviewing course (Murden *et al.* 2004). These identified deficiencies were correlated with third-year clerkship grades. Identified students as a group had significantly lower clinical grades than did matched controls. Those with identified paternalism and poor attitudes had significantly lower grades, those with poor process skills had lower grades that did not reach statistical significance owing to low numbers and those with shyness/communication troubles did not have appreciably lower grades. This suggests an ability within medical schools to teach or improve at least some students with problems in certain areas of professionalism. Interestingly, over the 6 years of this study, 6.7% of students were identified as having deficiencies, and 10% had dropped out or not graduated by study completion, similar to previously reported numbers of identified students.

One study showed that third-year medical school grades predicted poor professionalism ratings in internship, with no other medical school variables being independent predictors (Greenburg *et al.* 2007). A larger landmark study was a retrospective analysis of physicians from three medical schools who were disciplined by state medical boards (Papadakis *et al.* 2005). The odds ratio (OR) of these physicians having had significant reported unprofessional behaviour in medical school (compared with matched controls) was 3:1. The ORs were higher if the specific behaviour reported in medical school was severe irresponsibility (OR 8.5:1) or diminished capacity for self-improvement (OR 3.1:1).

Another study showed that the types of professionalism deficiencies noted in medical school were similar to those reported in physicians disciplined by the state medical board (Ainsworth and Szauter 2006). In this study, 73% of deficiencies reported in medical school were in the area of professional responsibility and integrity, and 14% in the area of insight and the pursuit of excellence. In physicians disciplined by the state medical board, a similar 77% were for problems with professional responsibility or integrity, and 20% for insight or pursuit of excellence issues. As opposed to the Papadakis study referenced above, however, the medical students and disciplined physicians came from different groups, and prediction of medical board actions in individuals was not implied.

Finally, it was reported that low professionalism ratings (four or less on a nine-point scale) in residency also correlated with state medical board disciplinary action (Papadakis *et al.* 2008). The OR was 2.2 in this study, and 1% of the group evaluated had a disciplinary action by the medical board.

In summary, several studies have shown that identified professionalism deficiencies as early as the first semester of medical school predict subsequent poor grade performance, poor professionalism ratings and state medical board disciplinary action. Only one of these (Murden *et al.* 2004) has shown any evidence that students with identified deficiencies can improve, although none of these studies reported specific remediation attempts. Thus, we are still left with the finding that 2 to 6% of medical students will have professionalism difficulties, and our ability to teach/improve these students is unclear.

Summary: can professionalism be taught?

There is evidence that, to some extent, the professionalism which is defined by a set of skills, knowledge, attitudes and behaviours can be taught. Effectiveness, though modest, of specific courses in these areas has been demonstrated, and some students identified early as having deficiencies have improved. Furthermore, there is virtually no literature evaluating remediation attempts. Since identification of the 2 to 6% of students who are most in need of remediation/learning professionalism has been shown to be achievable, much research is needed concerning remediation in this group. Until that research is done, there will be a large question mark as to whether professionalism can be taught to those most in need. One caveat to this concern is the presumption that professionalism is a dichotomous variable (present or absent). If professionalism is more reasonably considered a continuous variable, as has been suggested (Ginsburg *et al.* 2000, Hafferty 2000), then any movement in a positive direction on that continuum would be evidence that we are teaching professionalism.

Unfortunately, some of the evidence to date concerning movement on a continuum during medical school is in a negative direction. It has been well documented that there is a decline in empathy during medical training (Hojat *et al.* 2004). Certainly, the hidden curriculum and negative culture towards professionalism that exist to some extent in many medical schools can be pushing students in the wrong direction. It seems abundantly clear that much work must be done to improve these issues. Good role models need to be virtually ubiquitous among medical school faculty, which will require significant institutional support in the areas of faculty development, freeing up faculty to have time to teach (i.e. increased monetary support for education), devaluing unprofessional but lucrative faculty activity, reducing faculty and student stress and rewarding professional behaviour.

The bottom line is that professionalism can be taught. Unless admissions committees discover a way to completely weed out the 2 to 6% of students who seem to enter medical school with some degree of inherently unprofessional behaviours or attitudes, we may not be able to eliminate medical school graduates with some element of unprofessionalism when measured as a dichotomous variable. Good remediation studies have yet to be done in this group, however, so there is hope in that regard. In addition, what we can do is focus on teaching strategies of reflection, narrative and community and experiential service learning that have both theoretical and practical bases for success. We can greatly modify the environment that dominates the learning of professionalism, which is the culture of medical schools and academic medical centres. We can suggest that more elements of continuing medical education and accreditation be devoted to professionalism – for, as Hafferty points out, for all of their push towards improving professionalism, the American Association of Medical Colleges accreditation is for teaching the knowledge base of professionalism, not for producing more professional graduates (Hafferty 2000). Finally, we can make evaluation of professionalism as important in the medical school curriculum as the learning of the cranial nerves. As Hafferty also points out, in a very telling statement, if medical schools truly valued professionalism, Kaplan would teach it (Hafferty 2000). Are we teaching professionalism now? Yes we are, but in both positive and negative directions. Can we do a much better job? Yes, we likely can, but it will take a lot of effort in the areas noted above. Making this effort is crucial to the current international efforts to teach/improve professionalism among medical students.

References

Ainsworth M A, Szauter K M (2006). Medical student professionalism: are we measuring the right behaviors? A comparison of professional lapses by students and physicians. *Academic Medicine* **81**, S83–S86.

Archer R, Elder W, Hustedde C, Milam A, Joyce J (2008). The theory of planned behaviour in medical education: a model for integrating professionalism training. *Medical Education* **42**, 771–777.

Bennett A J, Roman B, Arnold L M, Kay J, Goldenhar L M (2005). Professionalism deficits among medical students: models of identification and intervention. *Academic Psychiatry* **29**, 426–432.

Boenink A D, de Jonge P, Smal K, Oderwald A, van Tilburg W (2005). The effects of teaching medical professionalism by means of vignettes: an exploratory study. *Medical Teacher* **27**, 429–432.

Brainard A H, Brislen H C (2007). Viewpoint: learning professionalism. A view from the trenches. *Academic Medicine* **82**, 1010–1014.

Coulehan J (2005). Viewpoint: Today's professionalism: engaging the mind but not the heart. *Academic Medicine* **80**, 892–898.

Cruess R L, Cruess S R (2006). Teaching professionalism; general principles. *Medical Teacher* **28**, 205–208.

Ginsburg S, Regehr G, Hatala R, *et al.* (2000). Context, conflict, and resolution: a new conceptual framework for evaluating professionalism. *Academic Medicine* **75**, S6–S11.

Ginsburg S, Regehr G, Lingard L (2003). The disavowed curriculum. Understanding students' reasoning in professionally challenging situations. *Journal of General Internal Medicine* **18**, 1015–1022.

Goldie J, Schwartz L, McConnachie A, Morrison J (2002). The impact of three years' ethics teaching, in an integrated medical curriculum, on students' proposed behaviour on meeting ethical dilemmas. *Medical Education* **36**, 489–497.

Greenburg D L, Durning S J, Cohen D L, Cruess D, Jackson J L (2007). Identifying medical students likely to exhibit poor professionalism and knowledge during internship. *Journal of General Internal Medicine* **22**, 1711–1717.

Hafferty F (2000). In search of a lost cord: professionalism and medical education's hidden curriculum. In D Wear and J Bickel (eds.) *Educating for Professionalism. Creating a Culture of Humanism in Medical Education.* Iowa City, IA: University of Iowa Press, pp. 11–34.

Hickson G B, Pichert J W, Webb L E, Gabbe S G (2007). A complementary approach to promoting professionalism: identifying, measuring, and addressing unprofessional behaviors. *Academic Medicine* **82**, 1040–1048.

Hojat M, Mangione S, Nasca T J, *et al.* (2004). An empirical study of decline in empathy in medical school. *Medical Education* **38**, 934–941.

Huddle T S (2005). Viewpoint: Teaching professionalism: is medical morality a competency? *Academic Medicine* **80**, 885–891.

Jha V, Bekker H L, Duffy S R, Roberts T E (2007). A systematic review of studies assessing and facilitating attitudes towards professionalism in medicine. *Medical Education* **41**, 822–829.

Joyner B D, Vemulakonda V M (2007). Improving professionalism: making the implicit more explicit. *Journal of Urology* **177**, 2287–2291.

Leo T, Eagen K (2008). Professionalism education: the medical student response. *Perspectives in Biology and Medicine* **51**, 508–516.

Mazor K M, Zanetti M L, Alper E J, *et al.* (2007). Assessing professionalism in the context of an objective structured clinical examination: an in-depth study of the rating process. *Medical Education* **41**, 331–340.

Moore G, Block S, Briggs-Style C, Mitchell R (1994). The influence of the new pathway curriculum on Harvard medical students. *Academic Medicine* **69**, 983–989.

Murden R A, Meier D E, Bloom P A, Tideiksaar R (1986). Response of fourth-year medical students to a required clinical clerkship in geriatrics. *Journal of Medical Education* **61**, 569–578.

Murden R A, Way D P, Hudson A, Westman J A (2004). Professionalism deficiencies in a first-quarter doctor–patient relationship course predict poor clinical performance in medical school. *Academic Medicine* **79**, S46–S48.

Papadakis M A, Arnold G K, Blank L L, Holmboe E S, Lipner R S (2008). Performance during internal medicine residency training and subsequent disciplinary action by state licensing boards. *Annals of Internal Medicine* **148**, 869–876.

Papadakis M A, Loeser H, Healy K (2001). Early detection and evaluation of professionalism deficiencies in medical students: one school's approach. *Academic Medicine* **76**, 1100–1106.

Papadakis M A, Teherani A, Banach M A, *et al.* (2005). Disciplinary action by medical boards and prior behavior in medical school. *New England Journal of Medicine* **353**, 2673–2682.

Parker M, Luke H, Zhang J, Wilkinson D, Peterson R, Ozolins L (2008). The "Pyramid of Professionalism": seven years of experience with an integrated program of teaching, developing, and assessing professionalism among medical students. *Academic Medicine* **83**, 733–741.

Phelan S, Obenshain S, Galey W (1993). Evaluation of the noncognitive professional traits of medical students. *Academic Medicine* **68**, 799–803.

Rees C E, Knight L V (2007). Viewpoint: The trouble with assessing students' professionalism: theoretical insights from sociocognitive psychology. *Academic Medicine* **82**, 46–50.

Self D, Olivarez M, Baldwin D (1998). The amount of small-group case-study discussion needed to improve moral reasoning skills of medical students. *Academic Medicine* **73**, 521–523.

Shrank W H, Reed V A, Jernstedt G C (2004). Fostering professionalism in medical education. A call for improved assessment and meaningful incentives. *Journal of General Internal Medicine* **19**, 887–892.

Smith L G (2005). Medical professionalism and the generation gap. *American Journal of Medicine* **118**, 439–442.

Steinert Y, Cruess R L, Cruess S R, Boudreau J D, Fuks A (2007). Faculty development as an instrument of change: a case study on teaching professionalism. *Academic Medicine* **82**, 1057–1064.

Stern D (1996). Values on call: a method for assessing the teaching of professionalism. *Academic Medicine* **71**, S37–S39.

Stern D, Cohen J, Bruder A, Packer B, Sole A (2008). Teaching humanism (medical student training) (Report). *Perspectives in Biology and Medicine* **51**, 495–506.

Stern D T, Frohna A Z, Gruppen L D (2005). The prediction of professional behaviour. *Medical Education* **39**, 75–82.

Stern D T, Papadakis M A (2006). The developing physician-becoming a professional. *New England Journal of Medicine* **355**, 1794–1799.

Swick H M, Szenas P, Danoff D, Whitcomb M E (1999). Teaching professionalism in undergraduate medical education. *Journal of the American Medical Association* **282**, 830–832.

West C P, Shanafelt T D (2007). The influence of personal and environmental factors on professionalism in medical education. *BMC Medical Education* **7**, 29.

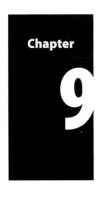

Chapter 9

Patient expectations from psychiatrists

Dinesh Bhugra and Susham Gupta

Editors' introduction

Two significant people at the core of any therapeutic encounter are the patient and the psychiatrist. The therapeutic encounter has the main purpose of establishing a diagnosis and devising a management plan. The encounter lies at the core of clinical judgement. When a patient comes to seek psychiatric help, especially from a psychiatrist compared with another member of the team, they come with certain expectations. They also bring with them their past experiences of their illness, their experience with other interventions and also their communicating styles. All of these in turn are influenced by their culture, gender, age, education and socio-economic status among other factors. They bring with them an expectation whereby they demand to know why something has gone wrong and what the psychiatrist can do to make it better for them. Their interest is in the illness which is affecting their social standing and functioning at different levels, whereas psychiatrists as doctors are interested in disease, which is about psychopathology. Thus, the patient expectations of the therapeutic encounter may well be at variance with those of the psychiatrist. This chapter highlights issues related to patient expectations of psychiatrists.

Introduction

Professionalism is described as the basis of medicine's contract with society. These components have been described elsewhere in this volume, and we will briefly look at them below. A major task of the psychiatrist as a clinician is to come up to and understand what the patients and their carers expect from them. The therapeutic encounter will be very strongly influenced by this, and the therapeutic engagement of the patient and carers will be dictated by what they expect from the psychiatrist.

The psychiatrist, like other doctors, has a responsibility to place the interests of the patient above his/her own, setting and maintaining standards of competence and integrity and providing expert advice to society. The nature of the psychiatrist–patient relationship in some settings is markedly different from that held by other doctors. In most countries, psychiatrists can deprive patients of their liberty and may recommend medium- or high-secure units, especially if serious crimes have been committed under the influence of mental illness. Furthermore, the possibility of breach of confidentiality always looms if the larger public or family are at risk. The psychiatrist–patient interaction thus becomes more unequal, and this is where an awareness of professional commitments and professionalism become significant.

Professionalism in Mental Healthcare: Experts, Expertise and Expectations, ed. Dinesh Bhugra and Amit Malik. Published by Cambridge University Press. © Cambridge University Press 2011.

Patients, especially if they are seeing a psychiatrist, irrespective of the setting, will often come with apprehensions and stigma attached to psychiatry and psychiatrists. However, this is far worse in some psychiatric conditions than others. Seeing a psychiatrist for the treatment of psychosexual dysfunction will have a different impact and expectations compared with a patient who is hypomanic and has florid psychotic symptoms. The patient is embedded in various cultures related to their culture of origin, age, gender, education and social and economic status, and some of these factors may take precedence over others depending upon the nature and the purpose of the encounter. In addition, the nature of the encounter will also vary depending on whether the patient is seeing the psychiatrist at home or on the ward, or whether this is the first contact or a follow-up. The expectations will fluctuate, but some core expectations will remain the same.

Review

There has been relatively little research carried out in the area of patient expectations of the therapeutic encounter. As a society evolves, the role of medical professionals and the expectations of patients change. Until the 1950s treatments were primarily random, and the doctor's role was to provide support in the form of allaying anxieties and providing clinical and emotional support. In the early years of the National Health Service in the UK, there was often little accountability to the tax-paying public; also, as a result of the medical services that people were used to paying for, there seemed to be a palpable sense of relief and generally lower patient expectations. This was also applicable to psychiatrists, whose primary role before the advent of medial treatments was to look after patients in mental asylums who had limited hope of improvement or of returning to a normal life. When the asylums closed and treatment moved to the community, the expectation was to keep patients well enough to be part of society. Patients also expected to be provided with a dignified existence as members of society, and thus they expected the mental health team to support them in order to achieve this aim. This also coincided with changes in mental health legislation to ensure that these patients in the community also received appropriate treatments when unwell. Psychiatrists thus had the unenviable dual role of healing as well as being able to restrict people's liberty and treat them against their will. Moreover, the integration of patients with society was often not smooth and they were often marginalized, which left them feeling disappointed, alienated and stigmatized. The psychiatrist–patient relationship thus became a forum where their frustrations could be played out. This was further complicated by the fact that sometimes the psychiatrist was the only mental health professional with whom they had a long-term relationship, often not by choice.

In the past few decades there has been a greater emphasis on the accountability of the medical profession. With the emergence of alternative medications and therapies, patients want to be reassured that they are being provided with the best available care. The Internet age has also made an enormous amount of knowledge available to doctors as well as to patients and their carers. Although all of this is primarily good, it can also lead to a divergence of opinion. Just as the expectations of patients and psychiatrists may differ at times, there are other important players in the arena – including the political establishment, the media, the legal system, the private healthcare providers and the pharmaceutical companies – who directly or indirectly influence this process.

In the United States, managed care programmes have provided physicians with financial incentives aimed at reducing the ordering of expensive tests and procedures, and this has raised concerns about patients' trust in their doctors (Levinson *et al.* 2005). The authors used a survey technique with 2765 subjects, and random scenarios of disclosure strategies were studied. Negotiations and addressing emotions in the disclosure were associated with best outcomes, and Black and Hispanic subjects were less likely to express satisfaction. The negotiation strategy reflected an approach that emphasized learning the patient's perspective, presenting the physician's perspective and finding an acceptable plan for both parties.

Addressing emotions encouraged the patient to express feelings and concerns and to share these concerns if conflict surfaced. Thus, it becomes obvious that it is possible to deal with responses in a pragmatic manner. The authors commented that it is possible for physicians to provide information, share concerns, deal with emotions and negotiate next steps effectively.

Patient expectations have been studied in primary care settings. McKinley *et al.* (2002) surveyed 3457 patients who had requested out-of-hours care. Patients were asked to fill in a satisfaction questionnaire. More than half the respondents were female. Patients who received care in line with their expectations were significantly more satisfied than those who did not. It is not surprising that the match or mismatch between the service patients hope for and the service they receive may then translate into levels of satisfaction with the service, whether it is in primary care or secondary care. The authors conclude that meeting or failing to meet idealized expectations of care is an important determinant of patient satisfaction. Therefore, in order to measure patient satisfaction in psychiatry it is important that expectations of care are studied.

Also in primary care, Keitz *et al.* (2007) noted that patients' expectations were met in the clinical encounter in two thirds of cases. Interestingly, expectations for medications and tests were met more frequently. In contrast, physicians acknowledged that in 45% of requests, tests would not have been ordered had the direct request not been made, and in 13% of cases they felt uncomfortable filling requests but nevertheless did so. The expectations in this study related to medication, tests and referrals to other agencies. Unmet expectations were explained satisfactorily by the physicians, with the provision of alternatives which were acceptable to the patient. Thus, these findings indicate that it is possible to negotiate even if the patient presents with certain expectations. Direct communication, as the authors conclude, affects the management of expectations. For physicians, learning how to effectively negotiate and respond to patient requests will certainly enable them to work with patients (and by extension with the carers) to develop stronger levels of therapeutic engagement. Keitz *et al.* (2007) recommend training doctors to negotiate effectively with patients and to respond to both appropriate and inappropriate demands and expectations. Their study also reflects changes in the doctor–patient relationship in the twenty-first century, where a sense of equal negotiation is apparent.

Laing (2002) points out that healthcare changes in the last quarter of a century have led to the reorientation of healthcare services around the patient, which has fundamental implications for healthcare providers and for challenging the dominance of healthcare professionals. Patient expectations are also likely to change according to their symptoms. Delgado *et al.* (2008) found, in a primary care setting, that expectations were high but depended upon the nature and severity of the complaints. In a primary care study from the UK, most patients wanted an explanation for their problems and had less desire for investigations and prescriptions (Williams *et al.* 1995). This may reflect a view that patients seek clarification, especially from someone who may be seen as wiser and more experienced. A similar finding from Taiwan indicated that patients base their evaluation of the therapeutic encounter on sophisticated expectations which vary according to social and demographic factors (Hsieh and Kagle

1991). Choice of physician has also been shown to be associated with increased satisfaction, again in primary care (Kalda *et al.* 2003). However, these authors also point out that other factors – such as the size of the practice, patient age and health status – also play a role. It is inevitable that expectations and the resulting satisfaction will vary according to the symptoms and the specialty that help is sought from. Korsch *et al.* (1968) noted that in paediatrics, a lack of warmth and friendliness on the part of the doctor, along with a failure to take the parents' expectations and concerns into account, a lack of a clear-cut explanation concerning the diagnosis and cause of illness and the use of medical jargon were important factors contributing to dissatisfaction. Thus, similar factors – inability to listen, lack of warmth, use of jargon and poor, garbled, incomplete or confusing explanations of diagnosis, aetiology, treatment plan and outcome – will all be apparent across several medical specialties along with psychiatry.

It is well known that the prevalence of psychiatric disorders is associated with socio-economic status which, combined with jargon-laced explanations, may alienate the patients and their carers in the therapeutic encounter. Understanding and managing patients' expectations are important in therapeutic engagement. We shall now look at what patients and carers expect of their psychiatrists.

Patient and carer expectations

Patients and carers expect psychiatrists, along with other members of the team, to be professional. Professionalism has the key attributes of primacy of patient welfare, principles of patient autonomy and social justice. Commitments to professional competence, honesty with patients, patient confidentiality, appropriate relationships with patients, improving quality of care and access to care, just distribution of finite resources, information, scientific knowledge, and maintaining trust and managing conflicts of interests are all important. A commitment to professional responsibility means that psychiatrists, like other physicians, work collaboratively in maximizing patient care, should be respectful of one another, participate in self-regulation and set standards for training and service. These standards, set by the American Board of Internal Medicine and the Royal College of Physicians in the UK, have already been widely accepted across specialties. The notions of patient autonomy, especially in the context of detained patients, require further deliberation and debate. Patients and their carers expect nothing less.

The very expectations that patients have of their psychiatrists were explored in focus groups at the Royal College of Psychiatrists in 2007. The groups comprised both carers and patients, and some preliminary findings have already been published (Bhugra *et al.* 2010). Contemporaneous notes were taken and a thematic analysis was carried out to explore the very themes. There were no real differences between the expectations of patients and carers, some of which are highlighted below.

Being knowledgeable

In the UK, psychiatrists are expected to have knowledge, not only in the field of psychiatry, but also in other related and relevant areas such as the justice system, capacity and how to assess mental capacity, the Disability Discrimination Act and its implications, the Human Rights Act, and so on. Combining biological, psychological and social approaches in order to identify aetiology and plan treatment are the core functions of the psychiatrist. Spiritual and cultural factors are becoming increasingly important in the demand for the provision of the holistic care which patients expect. Keeping up-to-date is one of the core attributes of professionalism. Patients expect their psychiatrists to have a lifelong commitment to reflexive learning, critical appraisal of the evidence and using this evidence to provide the most effective and acceptable service.

Being honest and approachable

Patients expect their doctors to be honest, and conflicts of interest need to be declared. This may be less of a problem in some healthcare delivery settings compared with others. In cultures and societies where kickbacks from private laboratories occur, the patients have the right to know why they are being referred to one laboratory and not another. Psychiatrists, like most doctors, are expected to be approachable and accessible. Accountability to society through its agents, such as regulatory bodies, can be related to being both honest and approachable. Being committed to high standards of healthcare delivery and high standards of personal behaviour are important. Patients have to believe that they can approach their psychiatrists and trust them.

Healing

Healing has been the central role of the medical profession since time immemorial. Healing includes alleviating or curing physical and psychological discomfort and helping the person return to his or her previous healthy state. Healing can also mean social, spiritual and emotional recovery. This wide concept of healing, especially in psychiatry, needs to be clearly understood and defined. This should reflect the changes in society and the development in medical sciences and the delivery of healthcare. Patients referred to psychiatrists may well have long-term conditions, and expectations of being cured can be unrealistic under these circumstances; part of the psychiatrist's role in such cases is to hold the patient's hope and deal with their and their family's anxieties. The role of the psychiatrist is central to the assessment of the clinical situation in the biopsychosocial framework and to working out a care plan in partnership with the patient whenever possible. With the increasing dependence on medications and various forms of therapies, the role of the psychiatrist is more one of an expert clinician who can guide and support the patient in making decisions regarding his or her care. He or she must also be able to maintain optimism while keeping realistic expectations.

Being ethical

Being an ethical practitioner was seen by the patients and carers as an important aspect of the practice of psychiatry. Ethical practice, high standards of personal behaviour and self-regulation are significant. The role of altruism in professionalism in the twenty-first century needs to be redefined. As clinical practice is becoming more consumer-oriented, it is inevitable that the definitions of altruism will vary, especially across different healthcare systems. In state-funded healthcare, altruism will have a different significance in comparison with a fully private healthcare system. Ethical practice also means that the individual practitioners follow several sets of ethics – those of the society, those of the profession and personal ones.

Emotional intelligence

Decision-making, whether in medicine or elsewhere, often requires not just knowledge and training, but also intuitiveness and experience. Much of the decision-making in a field like psychiatry involves emotional intelligence. Although efforts have been made to standardize delivery of care, patients expect a doctor to see beyond the illness and treat them as a whole. A patient expects the psychiatrist to be interested in their situation and provide an empathic, acknowledging and contained environment where he or she can talk about their most difficult experiences and emotions. Often the main complaints that patients have is the lack of opportunity to talk things through.

It is also important that the right people enter the profession in the first place. Suitability for a career in psychiatry could be assessed early on, with greater opportunities for 'tester' placements. Further training and experience can also improve a doctor's ability to develop existing skills. Better-quality patient feedback is another useful way of assessing these skills prior to entry or later on in training.

Communicating

Being a good communicator is at the heart of psychiatry. Psychiatrists need to communicate well not only with patients and carers but also with their teams on a close level and with society and the community on a more distant level. Using these skills can contribute towards reducing stigma, but at the patient level, better communication can lead to better rapport and trust. Conveying empathy and an understanding of the patient's experiences is essential. Keeping clear and accurate records and sharing information with team members and the patient are fundamental to the clinical relationship. Communicating with the society at large can also be helpful.

Sharing information

Sharing information at the right level with patients and carers about the diagnosis, management and outcome forms part of patients' expectations. Additional information written in simple terms that can be easily understood is often helpful. Sharing information within the bounds of confidentiality is important. Patients and carers made it very clear that they did not want their psychiatrists to be paternalistic, arrogant or patronising.

Being paternalistic

Medicine has historically been a paternalistic profession. This stems from a long-standing traditional role as a healer who aimed to take control of the situation and provide faith to individuals and families in times of uncertainty. It was also a way of trying to ensure compliance with treatments. Lack of knowledge of illnesses and treatments also meant that the patient was at the mercy/discretion of the doctor or healer. As a result, the doctor could potentially become patronising and even arrogant. As the main form of treatment delivery shifted from individuals to services provided by the state, this dynamic started to change. Codes of conduct also started to control professional behaviour. As a tax-payer, the patient became much more empowered as a purchaser of services. Given that more healthcare systems around the globe are now being provided by the state, healthcare professionals are becoming accountable to their citizens. This has also meant that medical services, including psychiatric services, have become part of the political agenda, as healthcare usually accounts for a sizeable portion of the gross domestic product in most developed countries. The media often use this as a political tool to attack governments as a way of demonstrating public control of resources. With increasing accountability and feelings of entitlement came the risk of unachievable, unrealistic expectations. The role of the healer has lost a certain amount of the public's and patient's trust, even though the quality of care provided is probably the best it has ever been. So what has changed and why? Part of the problem is the change in society's expectations and the emergence of the 'blame culture', which has been exploited by legal practitioners as well as the media. Furthermore, the medical services, especially psychiatrists, have fallen into the trap of becoming an instrument for the implementation of prescribed government policies which are often politically motivated and target driven. In addition psychiatrists may have promised a lot, but their failure to deliver has further alienated people. With a patient population which is generally disadvantaged, sidelined and hence distressed, it is not difficult to see how the psychiatrist can easily be viewed as a foe rather than an ally. Thus, often without adequate resources, psychiatrists find themselves in the unenviable position of being at the receiving end of patients', politicians' and the public's expectations.

Very few professions are as regulated as medicine, and psychiatry is no different. This is primarily for patient safety and to limit damage to the patients and the public. Part of the strategy is risk limitation and thorough risk assessments. Accountability for psychiatrists' actions is significantly higher than for the financial or legal sector. It is inevitable that mistakes in decision-making do happen, and these are often due to decisions that fail to reach optimum clinical or patient expectations and when the evidence base is not followed. However, even if mistakes cannot be totally eradicated, they can and should be minimized. Decision-making in psychiatry involves a complex series of judgements catering for each individual patient and clinical scenario (Bhugra 2008a, 2008b). There are various factors that can affect the ultimate outcome. However, society has become more litigious, which is not all bad and has probably made clinicians make decisions more carefully. However, on the flip side, as has been seen in the United States, there is a greater likelihood of defensive medicine being practised and of sticking rigidly to protocols and guidelines, which can reduce the degree of creativity and flexibility that is needed in a field like psychiatry. The media can be a potent factor in this equation. The repeated portrayal of mental health patients as a threat to the public, or untoward incidences – a direct result of the failure of the psychiatric services (often exploited by the political establishment) – have put significant pressure on psychiatrists in their decisions about positive risk management. This in itself sometimes influences the doctor–patient dynamic: these other external concerns are unlikely to be expressed or discussed, making the process look more punitive and reducing mutual trust.

Threats to professionalism were both internal, especially within the mental healthcare system, and external, arising from government policies related to encouraging consumerism, reducing investment and increasing control.

External threats noted by patients and carers were as follows: encouraging increased consumerism, especially by the politicians; the growth of new professions such as counselling and psychotherapy; the privatization of parts of the healthcare system; an emphasis on the 'dumbing down' of training by attempts to reduce the duration of training; and the impact of the 'celebrity culture', which was making psychiatry more fashionable, but only in private settings. Further research is needed to explore this.

Internal threats included bad practice, poor standards and limitation of models (of aetiology and management). Patients and carers wanted the professionals themselves, and through them the professional bodies, to take control and deal with threats to professionalism and the profession.

Patient expectations of the therapeutic encounter and what they want from their psychiatrist has to be seen in the context (i.e. service) within which it is being carried out.

Differences between outpatient and inpatient settings and between public and private settings will bring different issues to the actual consultation.

Characteristics of a good psychiatrist

A good psychiatrist is someone who is accessible, approachable and honest and who treats the patient as an equal partner in the therapeutic relationship. Keeping up-to-date with knowledge, developing and setting standards and ensuring that these standards are met and kept, being ethical and possessing excellent communication skills are the key characteristics which patients and carers expect of their psychiatrists.

With the ever-present stigmatization associated with the mentally ill, mental illness and psychiatrists, it is important that patients and psychiatrists have a common mutually agreed framework of standards and destigmatizing strategies. Patients and carers consider a good psychiatrist to be essentially a healer, communicator, listener and team player, adaptable and aware of the medical model but also aware of its limitations and gaps, someone who is able to synthesize information and convey it in an easily accessible and understandable manner, trustworthy, possessing the core values of respect and confidentiality and yet having a holistic approach (Bhugra *et al.* 2010). An understanding of the explanatory models held by the patient was seen as an essential attribute of good psychiatrists. Working with families, treating everyone with respect and avoiding personal prejudices wherever and whenever possible were identified as important components of professionalism. It would appear that the gulf between the patients' and carers' notions of professionalism and those of the professionals is non-existent, which is a reassuring sign.

Conclusions

There is a grave need for redefining the role of the healer and involving society to adapt to this. Healing in the form of 'curing' is outdated in many ways. Failure to cure is not a failure to care as long as the patient's best interests remain central to the therapeutic encounter. Unlike the traditional doctors of the past, modern psychiatrists depend on pharmacotherapy, a multidisciplinary mental health team and government policies (including mental health laws) in order to deliver care. It is now time to emphasize professionalism, which can clarify the psychiatrist's role and increase confidence. This would also mean being realistic about our expectations of society and would put the onus on us to strengthen the profession through internal support systems and introspective development. Work needs to be done to attract the best trainees to enter the profession out of respect for it. We would need to renegotiate the psychiatrist–patient relationship, reduce mutual distrust and build confidence. There is also a need to challenge the inaccurate portrayal of mental health, both in general terms and as a soft target for the media and politicians, primarily by dialogue and through the user movement. The patient must be able to see the psychiatrist as a caring professional who treats him or her with respect, provides medical guidance especially in times of crisis and can advocate on his or her behalf. Importantly, they should be able to engage in an honest dialogue based on knowledge and realistic expectations. This should be centred primarily around the best interests of the patient and not on external expectations.

References

Bhugra D (2008a). Decision-making in psychiatry: what can we learn? *Acta Psychiatrica Scandinavica* **118**, 1–3.

Bhugra D (2008b). Decision making by patients: who gains? *International Journal of Social Psychiatry* **54**, 1.

Bhugra D, Gupta S, Smyth G, Webber M (2010). Through the prism darkly: how do others see psychiatrists? *Australasian Psychiatry* **18**(1), 7–11.

Delgado A, Lopez-Fernandez L A, Luna J de D, Gil N, Jimenez M, Puga A (2008). Patient expectations are not always the same. *Epidemiology and Community Health* **62**, 427–434.

Hsieh M O, Kagle J D (1991). Understanding patient satisfaction and dissatisfaction with health care. *Health & Social Work* **16**, 281–290.

Kalda R, Pollustek K, Lembe M (2003). Patient satisfaction with care is associated with personal choice of physician. *Health Policy* **64**, 55–62.

Keitz S A, Stechuchak K M, Grambowb S C, Koropchok C M, Tulsley J A (2007). Behind closed doors. *Archives of Internal Medicine* **167**, 445–452.

Korsch B M, Gozzi E K, Francis V C (1968). Doctor–patient interaction and patient satisfaction. *Paediatrics* **42**, 855–871.

Laing A (2002). Meeting patient expectations: health care professionals and service re-engineering. *Health Services Management Research* **15**, 165–172.

Levinson W, Kao A, Kuby A M, Thisted R A (2005). The effect of physician disclosure of financial incentives on trusts. *Archives of Internal Medicine* **165**, 625–630.

McKinley R K, Stevenson K, Adams S, Manku-Scott T K (2002). Meeting patient expectations of care: the major determinant of satisfaction with out of hours primary medical care? *Family Practice* **19**, 333–338.

Williams S, Weinman J, Dale J, Newman S (1995). Patient expectations: what do primary care patients want from the GP and how far does meeting expectations affect patient satisfaction. *Family Practice* **12**(2), 193–201.

Chapter 10

Teams and professionalism

David W. Page

Editors' introduction

There are very few specialties in medicine where doctors do not work in teams. The skills required to collaborate and be a team player have been identified as a core and significant part of professional roles and capabilities. Within any team, each member has specific responsibilities related to their discipline and to the skills. In spite of that, the individual team member is answerable to their own (specific) specialist regulator or society, but the ultimate care of the patient and the contract with the society is with the team. The focus of any successful and well-functioning team is to deliver high-quality care which is cost-effective and emotionally accessible to the patients and their carers. As a surgeon, Page works with surgical teams but the lessons for psychiatric teams are broadly similar. The challenges of and to professionalism are related to changing public and patient expectations, increased costs, conflicts of interest and consumerism. Increased cynicism among medical students and reduced empathy can be explained by a number of factors. Medical socialization and derogation of patients by students and trainees tend to contribute to a sense of superiority which is unwelcome in teams. Using the aviation industry as a model, Page argues that one of the biggest barriers to teamwork is the issue of leadership – who leads and why. In an aeroplane or in a surgical operation the leader is clearly identified, but in psychiatry this may be more difficult. The notion of work groups versus teams is worth remembering. From vertical silos across specialties, a more horizontal approach is becoming increasingly evident. Both the structure of the team and the team processes are important in ensuring that a team works smoothly. Page points out that teams tend to fail because their members lack a common goal. Other reasons are poor selection of team members, lack of time and interest, poor cross-over skills and a focus on activities rather than outcomes. The essence of teamwork is the model used for crew resource management. Page makes some very useful suggestions to team members to enable them to work together effectively and co-operatively for the greater good of patients.

Introduction

A physician's role in society is equally that of healer and professional (Cruess *et al.* 1999). Both of these fundamental elements of a doctor's daily work are in jeopardy today. The interposition of complex technology between the patient and the physician weakens the healer's bond, while – at least in the United States – market forces and state and federal regulatory oversight impinge on the autonomy of the medical professional. Additionally, with increasing

Professionalism in Mental Healthcare: Experts, Expertise and Expectations, ed. Dinesh Bhugra and Amit Malik. Published by Cambridge University Press. © Cambridge University Press 2011.

restrictions on trainee work hours, a new paradigm is needed for the way physicians work together. This chapter will argue that a more effective way is 'true' teamwork.

Teams have been around for centuries, but healthcare teams are relatively new. They contrast with more familiar congenial work groups that constitute the basic units of all hospitals. As a high reliability organization (HRO), a well-run modern hospital consists of many interdisciplinary teams (Baker *et al.* 2006). Not surprisingly, this web of specialized aggregations of doctors, nurses, technicians and other allied healthcare workers often finds its members participating in more than one unit.

Twenty-first century healthcare is characterized by torrid cost escalation, increasing technical complexity and unmediated uncertainty. The depth and breadth of medical knowledge have surpassed any individual practitioner's ability to master a fraction of the total scientific database. In fact, today the very definition of illness hinges as much upon social and cultural constructs as it does on pathophysiology and thus opens up more content areas to physician scrutiny. And as the number of procedural skills that (interventional) physicians and surgeons are required to master continues to grow, the time available to train doctors has decreased with regulated work hours (DaRosa *et al.* 2003, Chung 2005). One might argue that patient safety may deteriorate if better methods of medical education and ways of providing care are not devised.

These challenges open up opportunities for an expanded role for teams in healthcare. This is not in the least because of the increased public awareness of medical errors as a consequence of escalating technical complexity in practice (Kohn *et al.* 2000). Eliot Freidson (1970a) states, '…the occupational organization of the work of one learned profession constitutes a dimension quite as distinct and fully as important as its knowledge, and that the social value of its work is as much a function of its organization as it is of the knowledge and skill it is said to possess.' Teamwork constitutes the new type of organization to which Freidson refers; the 'one learned profession' is medicine. Teamwork promises the ability to complete a task and create a 'product' beyond the capacity of any single individual working in isolation (Marks *et al.* 2001). It has been suggested (Frankfort *et al.* 2000) that one strategy medical education may use to achieve common goals is to reach out into the practice world and create new 'institutions of reflective practice'. This notion implies that there is inherent value in teamwork.

The integration of true medical teams into healthcare in several countries has occurred to varying degrees with different results. For example, North American surgeons have traditionally functioned independently while European surgeons often relieve one another in shifts in the operating room. Not surprisingly, in one US study (Halverson *et al.* 2009) the introduction of a curriculum in team training for surgeons resulted in only a 66% compliance rate 6 months after implementation. However, regardless of how medical professionals function, Freidson (1970b) reminds us of our responsibility as unique professionals: 'The occupation sustains this special status by its pervasive profession of extraordinary trustworthiness of its members. The trustworthiness it professes naturally includes ethicality and also knowledgeable skill.'

The challenges of professionalism

In the United States, the Accreditation Council for Graduate Medical Education (ACGME) has defined six competencies which form the basis of physician training (ACGME Competencies 2009). As one of the six competencies, professionalism seems to be the most resistant to definition. Professionalism may be defined as a conglomerate of separate elements such as honesty, empathy, reliability, self-awareness, competence and so forth (Braddock and Fryer-Edwards 2002). Another approach is to define professionalism as a comprehensive ethical construct with almost limitless boundaries. Alternatively, professionalism may be seen as perhaps a combination of the two, one of the six ACGME competencies that overlaps the others. Whatever the construct, all trainees and practitioners must bear in mind what Larkin (2003) admonishes: 'Virtue promotion may be thought of as a kind of moral vaccination against ethical pitfalls inherent in modern medical practice.'

Some of the most ethically challenging dilemmas facing doctors include perverse economic and contractual incentives, conflicts of interest between physicians and industry, terrible market-place competition among doctors, resource utilization reviews and the time-consuming struggle to maintain competence across an enlarging corpus of medical knowledge and technical skills. The erosion of professionalism in the United States is underscored by investigations into Medicare and Medicaid fraud, kickbacks to doctors disguised as consultation fees, questionable drug prescribing practices, questionable scientific research as a result of unhealthy associations between academia and the pharmaceutical industry, industry's influence on physicians' choice of medical devices and unscrupulous practices by medical insurance companies (Abelson 2006, Luo and Perez-Pena 2006, Meier 2006, Whitaker 2007).

Economic pressures from rising practice costs and decreasing reimbursement rates create conflicts in academia as well as in the private sector in the United States (Chervenak and McCullough 2001). In the words of Pellegrino and Thomasma (1997), 'When economics and entrepreneurism drive the professions, they admit only self-interest and the working of the marketplace as the motives for professional activity. In a free-market economy, effacement of self-interest, or any conduct shaped primarily by the idea of altruism or virtue, is simply inconsistent with survival.' In this regard vascular surgeons and interventional radiologists, for example, constantly step on each other's procedural (and financial) toes in areas such as occlusive carotid arterial disease. The merging of related clinical fields into specialty hospitals inures doctors to work together co-operatively on interdependent teams.

The beginning of professionalism: a medical student's first 'team'

In the presence of the cadaver

Teaching professionalism begins in the first year of medical school in the anatomy laboratory where learners collaborate in a stressful environment (Slotnick and Hilton 2006). Anatomists are confronted with the conundrum of fostering sensitivity to the donor (cadaver) while at the same time managing the challenges novice trainees face when attempting to cope with a dead body. In the anatomy lab the seeds of professionalism must be sown in the presence of this ambiguity. Warner and Rizzolo (2006) propose that, while photographs of nineteenth-century medical students playing cards with a cadaver suggest a profound lack of respect for donors, anatomists have struggled to inculcate in their students a degree of professional 'affective hardness'. Also, as knowledge of physiology, histology, biochemistry, immunology and genetics expanded, anatomists had to reinvent their curricula and themselves (McWorter and Forester 2004).

Recently, anatomy labs have been transformed into arenas where group learning and an emphasis on teamwork are fostered. According to Swick (2006), 'Teamwork has become an important practice model, and it will become even more crucial as scientific and technological advances continue rapidly to improve patient care, and so it is imperative that medical students gain experience in working collaboratively.' Commenting on students working together in the anatomy lab, Warner and Rizzolo (2006) noted that, 'When brought together in a focus group to discuss learning strategy, many students were surprised and grateful to learn of the diverse strategies and resources that other individuals or dissecting teams used to solve common problems.' In preparation for working on clinical teams, first-year students should be encouraged to 'pre-round' in the anatomy lab and to share 'structural variation' lists and debrief each other at the end of the lab session – all modern strategies used in the team management of patients (Page 2006). This sort of collaboration also sets the stage for the clinical years, where multiple 'hand-offs' or handovers (patient information transfers) are mandated by restricted duty hours and the emergence of a 'shift' mentality. This skill is important, as recent studies (Belenky *et al.* 2003, Charap 2004, Van Eaton *et al.* 2005) have identified information transfers (between clinical teams) rather than trainee fatigue to be a major source of medical errors.

However, the selection of applicants to medical school confounds efforts to foster a team-based approach to patient care. Students are selected in a process aimed at identifying intellectual and personality traits known to assure individual success (single-minded focus on self-preservation, insulation from outside distractions, studying in isolation, outworking the competition, etc.). Until the institution of reduced work hours, these highly motivated trainees logged endless hours caring for their patients. Their mantra was total patient ownership. Working independently they met the primary component of professionalism: *placing the welfare of their patients above their own interests.* They also honoured other components of professionalism, including setting and maintaining standards of knowledge and skills competence, personal integrity, demonstrating a humanistic dedication to patients with compassion and empathy, demonstrating sensitivity to the patient's age, gender, religion, cultural and sexual orientation and socio-economic status and demonstrating honesty, decency, integrity, duty, accountability and respect for others (ABIM Foundation *et al.* 2002, Van Eaton *et al.* 2005).

On the surface, moving to a clinical model of working in teams rather than alone ought to be a smooth transition. To a very real degree the elements of professionalism and the characteristics of successful teams are concordant. Both require a commitment to developing and maintaining cognitive and motor skills of the highest order, as well as dedication to the use of these skills to communicate a seamless series of patient information exchanges ('hand-offs'). Why, then, is true teamwork so difficult to achieve?

The natural history of medical student cynicism

To understand the inherent difficulty involved in creating real medical teams with members that trust each other (perhaps the most critical factor in teamwork), one must acknowledge the change in medical students' attitudes and behaviours – a negative ethical transformation (degradation of empathy) – as the student advances through the basic sciences and undertakes patient-oriented tasks. It is against a background of professional slips and ethical transgressions that we may comprehend the enormous task of team building and of improving communication skills in the hospital setting and in other healthcare areas (Sutcliffe *et al.* 2004). Thus, it is critical for us to understand a proposed barrier to medical students and trainees working in teams (Hebert *et al.* 1992, Rezler 1974, Testeman *et al.* 1996):

fluctuating cynicism in students progressing through medical school which often reflects a 'hidden curriculum'.

Two models explain medical student cynicism. The 'intergenerational model' states that students become cynical because of mistreatment suffered at the hands of abusive residents and faculty. The 'professional identity model' suggests students succumb to the harsh processes of medical socialization and remain cynical until they establish their own authority as they progress up the training hierarchy. Ethical erosion may emerge as derogatory slang or in the form of making fun of patients. However, it has been suggested (Wear *et al.* 2006) that many derogatory words and phrases reported by medical students were quoted (e.g. the hidden curriculum) from trainees and faculty members.

Philosopher John Morreall (1987) theorizes that humour used by trainees may fall into one of three categories. The 'superiority' theory first espoused by Aristotle explains that one laughs at another because one feels superior (e.g. the GOMER phenomenon: 'Get out of my emergency room' – a reference to physically offensive, disadvantaged patients, e.g. incontinent, poor hygiene, habitual malingering, etc.) (George and Dundes 1978, Leiderman and Grisso 1985). The 'relief' theory assumes that one laughs to release the pent-up nervous energy (accumulated while caring for sick patients). The 'incongruity' theory suggests that humour emanates from a disconnect (reversal) between expectation and what the joke actually says about a patient.

The issue of students derogating patients provides another potential role for teams. Modifying medical student behaviour is important because, as has been demonstrated (Papadakis *et al.* 2004), unprofessional behaviour is strongly associated with subsequent disciplinary action by state medical boards. Hafferty (2002) has documented that some students foresee a problem integrating altruism into their lives because of their personal belief that they are not obliged to do anything. To encourage collaboration among groups of medical students, individuals should be encouraged to evaluate each other. Cohen (1999) insists peer assessment is consistent with their future roles as participants in granting licences, delimiting hospital privileges and granting memberships to societies and referral networks.

Professions and the ascent of professionalism

A study by the American Association of Medical Colleges (AAMC Study on Professionalism 1998) revealed that 90% of medical students received some education in professionalism. A student's moral reasoning is often challenged in specific ways during the clinical years. Dilemmas include being asked to write notes that contain false information, to document physical findings the student did not personally identify or to silently observe a novice trainee perform a procedure knowing the novice was not adequately supervised. Again, these issues serve a hidden curriculum of ethically opprobrious content that the student is ill prepared to confront but nonetheless may begin to assimilate. Fortunately, teaching medical ethics is feasible and may improve a student's moral reasoning (Benbassat and Baumal 2004, Rose *et al.* 2005, Branch 2006, Weismann *et al.* 2006). In this regard, a student's cynicism decreases with progression through residency training.

What is a profession?

The public willingly enters into a social contract with doctors and other professionals and, in so doing, provides those professionals with certain liberties and restrictions. Of all professions, medicine is most heavily burdened with the responsibility of meeting the public's expectations, while remaining true to its avowal to adhere to the ethical demands of doing no harm, doing good deeds, recognizing patient autonomy and assuring social justice. The American College of Surgeons' Task Force on Professionalism has stated that 'all professions are characterized by four elements' (Gruen *et al.* 2003):

- A monopoly over the use of specialized knowledge
- Relative autonomy in practice and the privilege of self-regulation
- Altruistic service to individuals and society
- Responsibility for maintaining and expanding professional knowledge and skills.

As a member of a highly regarded profession, a physician must not only be an exemplary role model. The doctor must also demonstrate unswerving personal integrity and compassion. Treating patients with dignity and respect requires that the doctor listen past the demands of identifying clues to a differential diagnosis. Doctors must delve into the patient's personal sickness narrative within which the objective medical history is ensnared. Perhaps professionalism discovers its unique voice when crushed between the opposing forces of empathy and objectivism.

Specialists who succumb to the sanitized allure of becoming pure technicians have by definition defaulted on their professionalism. Primary care doctors who lapse into 'pill pushing' risk the same descent into apathy. Also, professionalism may impose long-term obligations on practitioners, especially when cure is no longer possible. End-of-life care requires the support of the patient and his or her family through the termination of supportive care. In this regard, in *The Death of Ivan Illyich*, Tolstoy (1981) describes how Ivan Illyich suffered horrible pain alone, ironically surrounded by his indifferent family and feckless doctors as his cancer metastasized and consumed him. The Russian judge would fare no better in many of our twenty-first century hospitals (Page 2007). Professionalism too often disappears when death dances with 'the elephant in the room', and doctors flee in horror from the shadowy image of their own mortality.

Collaboration: the new practice paradigm

In the healthcare arena, tension has always existed between a physician's traditional philosophy of self-sufficiency and the necessity of working co-operatively on interdisciplinary teams. In today's highly technological healthcare world, collaboration can be life-saving. Of course, the formation of teams may or may not improve clinical performance in all healthcare venues. And, as Pryor (2005) has suggested, effective collaboration depends on a number of factors.

Virtually all fields of medicine are in evolution. Interventional medicine and minimally invasive surgery require teamwork in order to succeed safely. To comply with the requirements of working in groups, if not in true teams, doctors must dismantle their preconceived notions regarding patient ownership. Physicians must become disease-centred.

The development of focused expertise in centres of excellence serves to reduce duplication of effort and services, improve communication among specialists and improve marketing strategies. Rather than the traditional department-based practices currently in vogue (surgery, gastroenterology, radiology, etc.), collaborative team-oriented practices would be disease-based (Pryor 2005). Ample evidence exists to demonstrate the value of co-ordinating patient care across disciplines such as critical care medicine and surgery in reducing mortality and morbidity (Young *et al.* 1997). Also, educational collaboration for trainees practising evidence-based medicine could involve a trainee, a medical librarian and a research co-ordinator, illustrating another aspect of the value of teamwork (Toedter *et al.* 2004).

The nature of teams

What constitutes a well-functioning team?

Each team member brings a unique set of cognitive, motor and behavioural skills to the co-operative effort. Differing cultural, social and educational backgrounds offer opportunities as well as barriers to teamwork. Prejudices and personalities add to the mix. Katzenbach and Smith (1993) state that the following interpersonal skills are vital to accomplishing the team's goals and common purpose: objectivity, giving and accepting helpful criticism, active listening, giving the benefit of the doubt and recognizing the interests and accomplishments of team members. Commenting on 'working together', Katzenbach and Smith (1993) continue, 'Every member of a successful team does equivalent amounts of real work; all members, including the team leader, contribute in concrete ways to the team's work product.' This is true whether the team involves a single discipline or is a 'multiple disciplinary' team.

For example, a surgeon will spend much of his or her professional time in the operating room, working with anaesthesiologists and various other members of the operating room support services. The same surgeon may also be part of a trauma service which includes surgical trainees, emergency department personnel, specially trained nurses, physician assistants and rehabilitation professionals. And, of course, the smooth running of the surgeon's office relies on a receptionist, a nurse, a practice manager and possibly others. But in a strict sense these units may or may not function as true teams. Similarly, a psychiatric team will have psychiatrists, trainees, psychologists, nurses, social workers and occupational therapists.

Immediately we run into one of the primary dilemmas that fomented the aviation industry's interest in and development of 'crew resource management', or CRM. One of the biggest barriers to teamwork is the issue of leadership (Helmreich *et al.* 1999). In a word, aviators discovered that the 'captain-of-the-ship' often listens poorly and is thus prone to making mistakes. It matters little if the 'ship' is an Airbus, an emergency department trauma bay or an operating room. The aviation industry and healthcare professionals who have adopted CRM quickly discovered that the key to improving professional performance resides in the contributions of the collective membership of the 'ship', whether those team members are co-pilots, navigators, surgical assistants, scrub techs or circulating nurses. In other words, one of the values of a team may be referred to as 'the wisdom of the group' (collective knowledge). However, that wisdom will only surface if it is accompanied by the ability to express one's opinion without regard to rank. Before we discuss how teams actually work, consider the differences between loosely knit collections of individuals and true teams.

Work groups versus teams

It is important to make distinctions among different collections of like-minded workers. Work groups may include executive committees, designated specialty work groups, ad hoc committees and other assemblies who do not meet the strict criteria of a team. Be they students, athletes or employees of an organization gathered to work together, 'feeling the chemistry' does not make them a true team.

Traditionally, medical specialties with hospital-based interventional suites formed silos or vertically integrated care units. Examples are psychiatry, gastroenterology, cardiology and pulmonary care units. These self-contained areas seldom interacted with each other. Today (despite efforts to integrate doctors more 'horizontally') when specialists consult each other, their professionalism often carries a little rust. Disparaging labels too frequently characterize whispered exchanges between members of the same specialty tribe as part of a hidden curriculum that contagiously infects the socialization of medical students and young physicians, and, in a way, breeds insider smugness. Improved patient safety will only be achieved when the attitude of physicians working together is one of mutual respect.

The way teams function

Successful teams share a common goal. Usually, teamwork begins with a mandate – there is a problem that cannot be solved by a single individual. The specific need arises from a 'performance challenge' (Katzenbach and Smith 1993). An example might be the need to accomplish a 10% reduction in re-admissions after inpatient psychiatric treatment. *Specific goals* create opportunities to generate *visible gains*, which motivate a team to continue to *improve its performance*. But improvement will not occur unless there is something to measure. That metric must be a product that could not have been produced without the contributions of every team member. Katzenbach and Smith (1993) describe six 'team basics'. Besides complete openness, honesty and the need to employ good communication skills, *the six basic components of team discipline are*:

- A small number of team members – fewer than 12
- Each team member must have complementary skills
- Each team member must share a common purpose and a common set of *specific* performance goals with the other team members
- Each team member must have a working approach that is agreed upon by other team members
- Each team member must hold other team members mutually accountable.

A small group of motivated individuals with strong leadership may go their own way with minimal cohesiveness and little more than general guidelines with which to solve major organizational problems. A good example is a hospital department run by a strong chairperson who leads by example and challenges his or her members to be innovative. Other groups such as 'promotion committees', with a less well-defined need for distinct leadership, also work effectively. But they are not teams. On this point Katzenbach and Smith (1993) state, 'Often open communication, constructive interaction, and reasonable accountability is all a small group requires to accomplish its nonperformance purpose. Many organizational forums, committees, and ad hoc groupings meet these needs effectively.'

Team processes

Whether managing a disruptive psychiatric patient on a ward or salvaging a multiple-injury trauma victim in the emergency room (accident ward), physicians multi-task using complex clinical skills over varying periods of time. Marks *et al.* (2001) describe *a recurring phase model of team processes* in which input–process–output relationships repeat themselves over a series of related cycles of work. These cycles are characterized by *periods of action* alternating with *periods of transition*. While the action periods involve activities aimed at accomplishing the team's specific goals, the transition periods are times of reflection, evaluation and/or planning for further activities. During both phases, *interpersonal processes* are monitored. These include conflict management, stimulating motivation, confidence building and effect management, including issues with cohesion, frustration and morale. Marks *et al.* (2001) further state, 'Whereas the transition and action processes have a natural temporal rhythm and relationship to one another, the interpersonal processes can work as an attribute or liability throughout goal accomplishment episodes.'

Why teams fail

Perhaps the most important reason teams fail is a lack of commitment to a common goal (Katzenbach and Smith 2008). The intent of designated 'teamwork' may have been too abstract. Physicians imbued with individualism and long trained in personal accountability – and embedded in a professional culture of 'blame and shame' when things go awry – may shrink back into the womb of self-sufficiency when asked to work with others. Some physicians are unable to place their reputation in the hands of their colleagues. For these individuals there is no trust, no willingness to share a common goal. In today's complex clinical world these individualists create havoc.

Of course, there are other reasons why teams do not work. Katzenbach and Smith (1993) list the following critical factors involved in team failure:

- The task does not require the vigorous time commitment of a team effort
- Team members were not carefully chosen
- Team members do not feel comfortable relying on others they deem 'different' or inferior
- Team members may lack cross-over skills
- Team members may lose interest in the performance goals
- Goals may have been based on *activities* ('Let's meet and discuss trainee promotions'), not *outcomes* ('Each of us will monitor three trainees to assure they place appropriate documents in their portfolios by the end of the month before our promotions committee meeting').

CRM: the essence of teamwork

To reduce the 'pilot error' aspect of air crashes, NASA convened a conference to identify the reasons for human mistakes in the cockpit. The reasons as alluded to earlier were failures of interpersonal communication, decision-making and leadership. Termed 'crew' resource management to emphasize the need for teamwork to improve aviation safety, CRM is an error management system designed to improve human performance by avoiding errors, 'trapping' errors and mitigating their impact (Helmreich *et al.* 1999). Remarkably, in the hospital environment it was not surgeons but rather anaesthesiologists who began to address medical errors by adopting CRM principles in the operating room (Howard *et al.* 1992, Gaba 2000, Sundar *et al.* 2007).

CRM matured through several iterations that increasingly emphasized briefing strategies, situational awareness and stress management. The value of providing similar training in all branches of medicine is obvious. For example, a survey performed by Grogan *et al.* (2004) after an 8-hour CRM course involving several specialties and hospital administrators revealed that 95% of participants felt that CRM would reduce errors in their practices. No doubt, if asked, a small number of doctors would side with a minority of pilots who describe CRM as little more than a charm school (Helmreich *et al.* 1999). Investigators confirm that pilots (in lock step with surgeons) share unrealistic attitudes regarding the impact of stressors on their performances. Individual swagger and absolute certainty negate the potential benefits of teamwork in improving patient safety. For example, improvements in quality of care with CRM include a significant reduction in errors in several emergency departments (Risser *et al.* 1999, Moray *et al.* 2002).

The fundamental elements of CRM include skilled interpersonal communication, situation awareness regarding one's physical environment and other team members, shared mental models, trust and support of team members and shared responsibility for success and failure. Not all doctors and allied health workers are effective team players. Therefore, it is time to educate medical students about teamwork early in their training.

The role of simulation in teaching teamwork

High-fidelity simulated environments are useful for providing a *briefing–simulation–debriefing* format for low-frequency crisis events such as cardiac arrest or unexpected massive intra-operative haemorrhage (Tsuda *et al.* 2009). In this protected setting, trainees may explore the emotional challenges of working with teammates and other healthcare workers through a volatile life-or-death event followed by immediate formative feedback from observers as well as participants. Besides avoiding patient harm while learning crisis management, teamwork may be integrated with other learning opportunities involving a wide range of competencies, such as obtaining informed consent and giving bad news.

Simulated patient scenarios offer trainees an opportunity to fail without consequences to patients. They bridge the chasm left in a medical training system characterized by potential team members who come from different educational backgrounds and medical disciplines and who seldom train together. Two types of medical team training programmes are primarily simulator-based or classroom-based (Baker *et al.* 2006). Two simulator-based programmes are the well-known Anesthesia Crisis Resource Management (ACRM) course and the Team-oriented Medical Simulation (TOMS). Classroom-based programmes include MedTeams™, Lifewings™ and Geriatric Interdisciplinary Team Training (GTT). Teamwork may also be taught employing role-play, leadership education, presenting a 'challenging case' scenario, using OSCE (objective standardized clinical encounters) and Web-based curricula.

The integration of professionalism and teamwork

How to be a good team member

The hallmark of professionalism is the willingness to place the obligation of caring for one's patients ahead of one's personal needs. Similarly, effective team members ask themselves how they can help their fellow team members. Attending to a patient's welfare or to a team member's needs constitutes selfless physician behaviour. Healthcare will only be elevated above the self-serving bugle calls of capitalism by medical practitioners who are morally grounded and committed to their patients.

It is instructive to complete this discussion of teams and professionalism by listing Herbert M. Swick's (2006) nine core attributes of medical professionalism. As you read the attributes listed below, reflect on how each component easily applies to teamwork:

- Subordinate one's own interests to the interests of others
- Adhere to high ethical and moral standards
- Respond to societal needs
- Evince core humanistic values
- Exercise accountability for themselves and for their colleagues
- Demonstrate a continuing commitment to excellence
- Demonstrate a commitment to scholarship and to advancing the field
- Deal with high levels of complexity and uncertainty
- Reflect upon actions and decisions.

Self-health: another role for teams in healthcare

An estimated 25% or more American surgeons are 'burned out' (Balch *et al.* 2009). The terrible cost of depression and depersonalization no doubt affects other healthcare practitioners and will increase as physician shortages force practitioners to work long hours (or more restricted work hours) in complex healthcare systems. It seems reasonable to assume that doctors who employ a shared mental model of what they wish to accomplish together may be better able to anticipate and avoid the emotional fall-out of modern practice. Teamwork and the support of team members offer an antidote to isolation and excessive rumination about practice events often characteristic of the behaviour of individual practitioners, as well as an opportunity for fatigue management (Hiatt *et al.* 1998, Howard 2004).

Katzenbach and Smith (1993) suggest, ' … credible team purposes have an element related to winning, being first, revolutionizing, or being on the cutting edge.' Thus, teamwork may reinvigorate healthcare workers by offering the opportunity to indulge in the excitement of discovering common goals. Finally, teams may serve the purpose of self-preservation by encouraging physicians to honour their ultimate fiduciary avowal – to work co-operatively for the greater good of society.

References

AAMC (1998). *Study on Professionalism.* AAMC Council of Academic Societies. www.amsa. org/meded/prof.cfm. Last accessed 2 April 2009.

Abelson R (6 May 2006). Respiratory equipment maker settles U.S. kickback charges. *New York Times.*

ABIM Foundation, ACP-ASIM Foundation, EFIM (2002). Medical professionalism in the new millennium: a physician charter. *Annals of Internal Medicine* **136**(3), 243–246.

ACGME (2009). *Competencies.* www.acgme.org. Last accessed 12 April 2009.

Baker D P, Day R, Salas E (2006). Teamwork as an essential component of High Reliability Organizations. *Health Services Research* **41**(4), 1576–1598.

Baker D P, Gustafson S, Beaubien J M, Salas E, Barach P (2006). Medical team training programs in health care. *Advances in Patient Safety* **4**, 253–267.

Balch C M, Freischlag J A, Shanafelt T D (2009). Stress and burnout among surgeons: understanding and managing the syndrome and avoiding the adverse consequences. *Archives of Surgery* **144**(4), 371–376.

Belenky G, Wesensten N J, Thorne DR, *et al.* (2003). Patterns of performance degradation and restoration during sleep deprivation and subsequent recovery: a sleep dose response study. *Journal of Sleep Research* **12**, 1–12.

Benbassat J, Baumal R (2004). What is empathy, and how can it be promoted during clinical clerkships? *Academic Medicine* **79**(9), 832–839.

Braddock R L S, Fryer-Edwards K A (2002). Using the American Board of Internal Medicine's "Elements of Professionalism" for undergraduate ethics education. *Academic Medicine* **77**(6), 523–531.

Branch W (2006). Teaching respect for patients. *Academic Medicine* **81**(5), 463–467.

Charap M (2004). Reducing resident work hours: unproven assumptions and unforeseen outcomes. *Annals of Internal Medicine* **140**, 814–815.

Chervenak F A, McCullough L B (2001). The moral foundation of medical leadership: the professional virtues of the physician as fiduciary of the patient. *American Journal of Obstetrics and Gynecology* **184**(5), 875–880.

Chung R S (2005). How much time do surgical residents need to learn operative surgery? *American Journal of Surgery* **190**, 351–353.

Cohen J J (1999). Measuring professionalism: listening to our students. *Academic Medicine* **74**(9), 1010.

Cruess R L, Cruess S R, Johnson S E (1999). Renewing professionalism: an opportunity for medicine. *Academic Medicine* **74**, 878–884.

DaRosa D A, Bell R H, Dunnington G L (2003). Residency program models, implications, and evaluation: results of a think tank consortium on resident work hours. *Surgery* **133**(1), 13–23.

Frankfort D M, Patterson M A, Konrad T R (2000). Transforming practice organizations to foster lifelong learning and commitment to medical professionalism. *Academic Medicine* **75**(7), 708–717.

Freidson E (1970a). *Profession of Medicine: a Study of the Sociology of Applied Knowledge.* Chicago: The University of Chicago Press, p. xi.

Freidson E (1970b). *Profession of Medicine: a Study of the Sociology of Applied Knowledge.* Chicago: The University of Chicago Press, p. xv.

Gaba D M (2000). Anesthesia as a model for patient safety in health care. *British Journal of Medicine* **320**, 785–788.

George V, Dundes A (1978). The Gomer: a figure of American hospital folk speech. *Journal of American Folklore* **91**, 568–581.

Grogan E L, Stiles R A, France D J, *et al.* (2004). The impact of aviation-based teamwork training on the attitudes of health-care professionals. *Journal of the American College of Surgery* **199**, 843–848.

Gruen R L, Arya J, Cosgrove E M *et al.* (2003). American College of Surgeons' Task Force on Professionalism. Professionalism in surgery.

Journal of the American College of Surgeons **197**(7), 605–608.

Hafferty F W (2002). What medical students know about professionalism. *The Mount Sinai Journal of Medicine* **69**(6), 385–396.

Halverson A L, Anderson J L, Anderson K *et al.* (2009). Surgical team training. *Archives of Surgery* **144**(2), 107–112.

Hebert P C, Meslin E M, Dunn E V (1992). Measuring the ethical sensitivity of medical students: a study at the University of Toronto. *Journal of Medical Ethics* **18**, 142–147.

Helmreich R L, Merritt A C, Wilhelm J A (1999). The evolution of Crew Resource Management training in commercial aviation. *The International Journal of Aviation Psychology* **9**(1), 19–32.

Hiatt H H, Barnes B A, Brennan T A, *et al.* (1998). Special report: a study of medical injury and medical malpractice. *New England Journal of Medicine* **321**(7), 480–484.

Howard D L (2004). Do regulations limiting resident work hours affect patient mortality? *Journal of General Internal Medicine* **19**, 1–7.

Howard S K, Gaba D M, Fish M B, *et al.* (1992). Anesthesia Crisis Resource Management training: teaching anesthesiologists to handle critical incidents. *Aviation, Space, and Environmental Medicine* **63**(9), 763–770.

Katzenbach J R, Smith D K (1993). *The Wisdom of Teams: Creating the High-Performance Organization*. New York: HarperCollins Publishers, Inc.

Katzenbach J R, Smith D K (2008). *The Discipline of Teams*. Boston: Harvard Business School.

Kohn L T, Corrigan J M, Donaldson M S (2000). *To Err is Human: Building a Safer Health System*. Washington, DC: Committee on Quality of Health Care in America. Institute of Medicine. National Academy Press.

Larkin G L (2003). Mapping, modeling, and mentoring: charting a course for professionalism in graduate medical education. *Cambridge Quarterly of Healthcare Ethics* **12**, 167–177.

Leiderman D B, Grisso J A (1985). The Gomer phenomenon. *Journal of Health and Social Behavior* **26**, 222–232.

Luo M, Perez-Pena R (6 June 2006). U.S. assails Albany's efforts on Medicaid fraud. *New York Times.*

Marks M A, Mathieu J E, Zacarro S J (2001). A temporally based framework and taxonomy of team processes. *Academy of Management Review* **26**(3), 356–376.

McWorter D L, Forester J P (2004). Effects of an alternative dissection schedule on gross anatomy laboratory practical performance. *Clinical Anatomy* **17**, 144–148.

Meier B (22 September 2006). Federal officials scrutinizing company payments to doctors. *New York Times.*

Moray J C, Simon R, Jay G D, *et al.* (2002). Error reduction and performance improvement in the emergency department through formal teamwork training: evaluation results of the MedTeams Project. *Health Services Research* **37**(6), 1553–1580.

Morreall J (1987). *The Philosophy of Laughter and Humor*. Albany: State University of New York Press, pp. 3–6.

Page D W (2006). Professionalism and team care in the clinical setting. *Clinical Anatomy* **19**, 468–472.

Page D W (2007). Modern lessons from Tolstoy's The Death of Ivan Illyich. *Journal of Palliative Medicine* **10**(1), 249–251.

Papadakis M A, Hodgson C S, Teherani A, Kohatsu N D (2004). Unprofessional behavior in medical school is associated with subsequent disciplinary action by a state medical board. *Academic Medicine* **79**(3), 244–249.

Pellegrino E D, Thomasma D C (1997). *Helping and Healing*. Washington, DC: Georgetown University Press.

Pryor A D (2005). Surgical evolution: collaboration is the key. *Archives of Surgery* **140**, 237–240.

Rezler A G (1974). Attitude changes during medical school: a review of the literature. *Journal of Medical Education* **49**, 1023–1030.

Risser D T, Rice T T, Salisbury M L, *et al.* (1999). The potential for improved teamwork to reduce medical errors in the emergency department. *Annals of Emergency Medicine* **34**(3), 373–383.

Rose G L, Rukstalis M R, Schuckit M A (2005). Informal mentoring between faculty and medical students. *Academic Medicine* **80**(4), 344–348.

Slotnick H B, Hilton S R (2006). Proto-professionalism and the dissecting laboratory. *Clinical Anatomy* **19**, 429–436.

Sundar E, Sundar S, Pawlowski J *et al.* (2007). Crew Resource Management and team training. *Anesthesiology Clinics* **25**, 283–300.

Sutcliffe K M, Lewton E, Rosenthal M M (2004). Communication failures: an insidious contributor to medical mishaps. *Academic Medicine* **79**(2), 186–194.

Swick H M (2006). Medical professionalism and the clinical anatomist. *Clinical Anatomy* **19**, 393–402.

Testeman J K, Morton K R, Loo L K, Worthley J S, Lamberton H H (1996). The natural history of cynicism in physicians. *Academic Medicine* **71**(10), s43–s45.

Toedter L J, Thompson L L, Rohatgi C (2004). Training surgeons to do evidence-based surgery: a collaborative approach. *Journal of the American College of Surgery* **199**, 293–299.

Tolstoy L (1981). *The Death of Ivan Illyich*. New York: Bantam Books.

Tsuda S, Scott D, Doyle J, Jones D (2009). Surgical skills training and simulation. *Current Problems in Surgery* **46**(4), 261–372.

Van Eaton E G, Horvath K D, Pellegrini C A (2005). Professionalism and the shift mentality: how to reconcile patient ownership with limited work hours. *Archives of Surgery* **140**, 230–235.

Warner J H, Rizzolo L J (2006). Anatomical instruction and training for professionalism from the 19th to the 21st centuries. *Clinical Anatomy* **19**, 403–414.

Wear D, Aultman J M, Varley J D, Zarconi J (2006). Making fun of patients: medical student's perceptions and use of derogatory and cynical humor in clinical settings. *Academic Medicine* **81**(5), 454–462.

Weissmann P F, Branch W T, Gracey C F, *et al.* (2006). Role modeling humanistic behavior: learning bedside manner from the experts. *Academic Medicine* **81**(7), 661–667.

Whitaker B (4 March 2007). The week: medical center faces federal inquiry. *New York Times*.

Young G J, Charns M P, Daley J, Forbers M G, Henderson W, Khuri S F (1997). Best practices for managing surgical services: the role of cooperation. *Health Care Management and Research* **22**(4), 72–81.

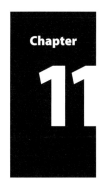

Chapter

11

New professionalism

Donna J. Schmutzler and James W. Holsinger, Jr

Editors' introduction

In some parts of the world, the deprofessionalization of medicine has been attributed to political imperatives, increased external control, levelling off of the doctor–patient relationship with patients having increased knowledge of their conditions, and nurse and psychologist prescribing, among other factors. It is important that while the profession decides and develops new definitions of professionalism, the definitions and causes of deprofessionalization be revisited and appropriate actions be put in place. Schmutzler and Holsinger provide an overview, arguing that professionalism can provide continuity and aid healthcare providers in defining values and supporting them. The values attributed to professionalization define healthcare providers and influence the way in which they work and deliver services. Abuse of power, arrogance, greed, misrepresentation, lack of conscientiousness, impairment due to illness or addictions and conflict of interest are the factors which may play a role in demoralizing healthcare professionals and subsequently lead to deprofessionalization. Improvements in the curriculum can cover some of these issues. However, healthcare values related to professional autonomy, patient autonomy, patient advocacy, consumer sovereignty, access to care and assurance of quality of care should be seen as core components of professionalism. Schmutzler and Holsinger redefine the values listed above in light of societal changes in the twenty-first century. They point out that instrumental values such as personal responsibility, social solidarity, social advocacy, provider autonomy, consumer sovereignty and personal security are all important concepts. The relationship between the physician on the one hand, and the society, the patient and the healthcare system on the other, is worth remembering.

Introduction

The healthcare professions have evolved over time, and consequently professional responsibilities have changed and become more technical in nature. Within the medical/social sciences and educational communities, the professions have been diligent in adapting to the transforming environment over the course of generations. Professionalism has a long history of being based on a defined set of values, and during the twentieth century professional autonomy was clearly the most important value among the healthcare professions, particularly among physicians (Holsinger and Beaton 2006). A century ago, Flexner (1910) aptly stated that '[n]o members of the social order are more self-sacrificing than the true physicians.' However, while addressing the students at the Harvard Medical School in 1927, Francis W. Peabody noted, 'The most common criticism made at present by older

Professionalism in Mental Healthcare: Experts, Expertise and Expectations, ed. Dinesh Bhugra and Amit Malik. Published by Cambridge University Press. © Cambridge University Press 2011.

practitioners is that young graduates have been taught a great deal about the mechanism of disease, but very little about the practice of medicine – or, to put it bluntly, they are too "scientific" and do not know how to take care of patients' (Peabody 1927). Thus, although major advancements in healthcare have occurred over the past 70 years, the emphasis on professionalism in its various guises has been pervasive, even in these times of physician dissatisfaction. The supremacy of predominantly physician-focused values such as professional autonomy has been supplanted by societal and patient-focused values such as fairer access to healthcare. The US healthcare system, like many others, is in the midst of reshaping some values and developing new ones to meet the needs of the healthcare environment for a new century (Priester 1992). With the passing of time, some professional values may become obsolete while others may be deemed invaluable. Professionalism, a time-honoured value, is being redefined to meet the needs of the twenty-first century, with the result that a new professionalism is coming into being.

The practice of professionalism

The practice of professionalism can provide continuity and enable healthcare providers to assist their colleagues and patients during a time of shifting professional values. Psychiatric educators are actively reviewing both materials and venues in order to determine the appropriate means of assisting healthcare providers during a time of change (Weiss Roberts *et al.* 2006). Continuing education activities directed towards practitioner professionalism provide the opportunity for practitioners to develop new ways of demonstrating professionalism in the workplace. Attention to professionalism as an important value in healthcare practice during the twenty-first century comes at a time of discontent for many physicians. 'Physicians, individually and collectively, have felt threatened and besieged' from different directions (Swick 2007). According to Holsinger and Beaton (2006), some factors causing dissatisfaction in this profession include: (1) loss of autonomy; (2) emergence and growth of managed care models; (3) increased specialization; (4) the medical liability crisis; (5) differences in physician and healthcare system expectations; and (6) decline in personal wellbeing.

Stevens (2002) noted that 'dominant explanations of the history of the medical profession during the past century have shaped public and professional attitudes in ways that are restrictive and unhelpful,' which can result in frustration. Rather than resist change, it is more productive to acknowledge, accept and actively participate in the change (Swick 1998). Providers and educators have the opportunity to participate in the development of the twenty-first century healthcare system based on an appropriate healthcare practitioner value system. In the process, the various healthcare professions will be renewed in an exciting and rewarding manner. The renewed interest in professionalism is a result of various factors, including physician discomfort, feeling of alienation, intrusion of external forces (including government and managed care organizations), medical practice changing from a professional model to a business model, defining the profession of medicine and erosion of societal responsibility of the underinsured and uninsured (Swick *et al.* 2006). According to Stevens (2002), the meaning of professionalism has changed such that, in the United States, the basic concepts of the profession of medicine need to be renegotiated. The gulf between the medical community and other entities, such as government or managed care organizations, must move away from conflict by healthcare practitioners focusing on the highest goals of society, such as universal healthcare (Stevens 2002).

Organizations in the United States such as the American Board of Internal Medicine (ABIM), the Accreditation Council for Graduate Medical Education (ACGME), the ABIM

Table 11.1 *Medical Professionalism in the New Millennium: A Physician Charter*

Preamble	Professionalism is the basis of medicine's contract with society
Fundamental principles	Professional commitments
Primacy of patient welfare	Professional competence
Patient autonomy	Honesty with patients
Social justice	Patient confidentiality
	Maintaining appropriate relations
	with patients
	Improving quality of care
	Just distribution of finite resources
	Scientific knowledge
	Maintaining trust by managing
	conflicts of interest
	Professional responsibilities

Source: ABIM Foundation *et al.* (2004).

Foundation, the American College of Physicians (ACP) Foundation, as well as the European Federation of Internal Medicine (EFIM), are all working to promote professionalism in medicine. Their efforts are equally applicable to the other healthcare professions. Although the traditional patient-focused Hippocratic Oath will continue to have validity, new documents are being developed to reflect the current realities of healthcare practice. The ABIM Foundation, ACP-ASIM Foundation and EFIM collaborated to publish *Medical Professionalism in the New Millennium: A Physician Charter* (ABIM Foundation *et al.* 2002); this presents the fundamental principles and professional responsibilities of today's physicians, which are applicable to other healthcare providers (Table 11.1). The document's preamble states that 'professionalism is the basis of medicine's contract with society. It demands placing the interests of patients above those of the physician …' (ABIM Foundation *et al.* 2002). The charter was developed in the interest of physicians reaffirming their 'active dedication to the principles of professionalism … intended to encourage such dedication and to promote an action agenda for the profession of medicine that is universal in scope and practice' (ABIM Foundation *et al.* 2002). As of 2003, the Physician Charter has been overwhelmingly endorsed by a total of 90 national and international organizations, including medical schools, certifying boards and professional societies (Blank *et al.* 2003). The Physician Charter is a valuable aid to understanding physician professionalism, but it is important to move beyond the charter to 'embrace the ideals, the genuine sense of selfless act, and the deep commitment to patients that have for so long epitomized the highest values of medicine' (Swick *et al.* 2006).

Professionalism values

The world is becoming more complex in the twenty-first century; the healthcare system is no different, as significant advancements have been made in science and technology. Dissatisfaction can lead to poor clinical management, patient dissatisfaction and a professionalism gap 'between the professional values espoused by the medical community and those demanded by society, patients, managers, and economic forces' (Holsinger and Beaton 2006). Thus, a consequence of this complexity is the loss of professional autonomy, which impacts feelings of self-worth and satisfaction of physicians and other healthcare practitioners (Holsinger and Beaton 2006). The values of professionalism define healthcare practitioners and their work. These values are the moral foundation of the healthcare community when they are focused on caring for the members of society. In previous years, physicians practised the values of professionalism, such as advocacy and service, while caring for patients through the use of a specialized body of knowledge, setting and maintaining high standards and meeting society's needs (Swick 1998). The American healthcare system currently functions within a system which emphasizes 'profit, competition, responsibility to stakeholders, services driven by the market, standards set by external forces, consumerism, short-term goals, and giving society what it thinks it wants' (Swick 1998). Thus, the current emphasis has been placed on the requirements of the healthcare system rather than on the needs of the patient.

The ABIM (2001) has defined seven issues that diminish professionalism in the medical community: (1) abuse of power is demonstrated during interactions with colleagues, patients and others by sexual harassment and through breaches of confidentiality; (2) arrogance is demonstrated through an inability to empathize with the patient, through removal of self-doubt and in visions of grandeur; (3) greed may be financial in nature and compromise values such as compassion, integrity and generosity as well as the physician–patient relationship; (4) misrepresentation may occur in the submission of fraudulent insurance claims; (5) impairment may be mental or alcohol- and drug-related; (6) lack of conscientiousness is incompatible with the quintessence of professionalism and is demonstrated through habitual inattention to professional responsibilities; and (7) conflicts of interest strike at the core of professionalism, occurring when self-interest outweighs patient interests, and can include self-referral of patients and the acceptance of gifts.

Academia has played an active role in the decline of professionalism by alienating patients and increasing the number of specialty areas within an ever more complex healthcare system that lacks altruism (Swick 1998). Owing to a decline in professional behaviour exhibited by physicians and medical students, professionalism has become a popular topic in medical journals and schools of medicine (Humphrey 2008). In recent years, medical schools have adapted the curriculum in order to assist the physicians of the twenty-first century to understand the value of professionalism.

Stevens (2002) states that professionalism has taken on an array of meanings, reflected through the need to teach virtues and warnings against personal corruption. 'Professionalism, it seems can no longer be taken for granted as a core of behavioral expectations that are inherent in becoming a physician' (Stevens 2002). Therefore, professionalism must be a focus in the academic setting and must be taught in such a way that, when physicians graduate, they enter the workforce committed to promoting the wellbeing of their patients, not only through the science of medicine but also though the art of medicine (Swick 1998) and 'grounded in the long-standing values of medicine' (Swick 2007). For many years professionalism has been an important, but largely ignored, aspect of a physician's ability to provide effective care to patients. Renee C. Fox (1990), a medical sociologist, states,

[F]ailing to recognize that in disjoining the art and science of medicine, we are pulling asunder technical competence and empathic caring…. [E]ach curriculum reform has been triggered by another prise de conscience about an excessive emphasis on the biological and technical aspects of medicine, at the expense of its psychological and humanistic components…. Over the last three decades, in their search for new formulas, North American medical schools have moved in seriatim from psychiatry, to psychosomatic medicine, to social and behavioral science, to community medicine, to bioethics, to the humanities.

Thus, Fox called for a reform of physician education in an effort to bring balance into their understanding of their professional role.

In developing curriculum materials on professionalism, various resources should be utilized so that the objectives are met and students find meaning in the courses. Resources can include information from professional organizations and/or professional boards and articles in professional journals. There are two distinct voices heard in the healthcare literature regarding professionalism. The first of these is the traditional view of professionalism, with the understanding that it develops over time as core values are inculcated. The second voice states that as structural changes in healthcare occur over time, an accompanying change in standards does not mean that the importance of professionalism has been lessened (Hafferty 2006). While studying at the University of Chicago Pritzker School of Medicine, Leo and Eagen (2008) raised issues concerning the way in which professionalism is taught and how the curriculum might be improved, and they identified issues that they believe detracted from their education on professionalism. Professionalism needs to focus on how to act in a professional manner. Students may gain a better perspective on professionalism if they are given positive rather than negative examples of the desired behaviours. Role-playing physician–patient encounters is one approach. There is often an erroneous belief by the faculty that students lack professionalism and thus they are being taught to 'be good people'. The students, on the other hand, believe their education needs to focus on teaching them how to be 'good physicians'. Owing to the length and depth of the curriculum, students question whether a curriculum which teaches students such things as how to dress professionally and act appropriately is justified. Students are also confused and frustrated by the double standard of 'do as I say, not as I do' when they witness faculty members, attending physicians and residents behaving in an unprofessional manner. As a result, students gain the impression that professionalism is a value taught to them but not practised by their mentors (Swick 2007). It should be noted that female psychiatrists were more interested in ethics training than their male counterparts during medical school and residency training (Weiss Roberts *et al.* 2006).

Improvements to the curriculum on professionalism include clarification to students on why professionalism is important to physicians, a focus on what comprises professional behaviour and exposure to positive role models (Leo and Eagen 2008).

Frameworks of professionalism

During the last few decades of the twentieth century, various professional organizations as well as other individuals considered the key components of professionalism, both as a value in and of itself, as well as considering it as an overarching framework governing the lives of healthcare practitioners.

Governing council frameworks

The ABIM, ACGME, ABIM Foundation and ACP Foundation, as well as EFIM, have been working separately or in partnership with one another to define and promote professionalism. The ACGME, a private, non-profit council established in 1981 for the purpose of evaluating and accrediting medical residency programmes in the United States, developed six competencies, including patient care, medical knowledge, practice-based learning and improvement, systems-based practice, professionalism and interpersonal and communication skills required for the practice of medicine (ACGME 2003). The professionalism competency is expressed through demonstrating 'a commitment to carrying out professional

Table 11.2 Priester's framework of healthcare values

Former values	Proposed values framework	
	Essential values	Instrumental values
Professional autonomy	Fair access	Personal responsibility
Patient autonomy	Quality	Social solidarity
Consumer sovereignty	Efficiency	Social advocacy
Patient advocacy	Respect for patients	Provider autonomy
Access to care	Patient advocacy	Consumer sovereignty
Assurance of quality of care		Personal security of care

Source: Priester (1992).

responsibilities, adherence to ethical principles, and sensitivity to a diverse patient population' (ACGME 2003). The ACGME lists the following aspects of professionalism which should be demonstrated by physicians:

- Respect, compassion, and integrity; a responsiveness to the needs of patients and society that supersedes self-interest; accountability to patients, society, and the profession; and a commitment to excellence and on-going professional development
- Commitment to ethical principles pertaining to provision or withholding of clinical care, confidentiality of patient information, informed consent, and business practices
- Sensitivity and responsiveness to patients' culture, age, gender, and disabilities (ACGME 2003).

The ACGME and the American Board of Medical Specialties (ABMS) have developed an assessment tool entitled *ACGME Competencies: Suggested Best Methods for Evaluation* that can be used to assess six competencies, including professionalism (ACGME 2000). This model and its assessment tool provide a significant approach to the development of a model of professionalism that can be introduced into postgraduate medical education.

Priester's framework of healthcare values

In 2006 Holsinger and Beaton proposed adapting Priester's values framework, developed in anticipation of the proposed Clinton healthcare reforms, as professional values for a new generation of physicians. Priester (1992) identified six influential values which had been dominant in the twentieth century: (1) professional autonomy; (2) patient autonomy; (3) consumer sovereignty; (4) patient advocacy; (5) access to care; and (6) assurance of quality of care (Table 11.2). He discerned that no specifically agreed set of values has existed that would allow the development of a coherent framework for the healthcare system. 'In practice, professional autonomy has been the most dominant value, while access to care has been subordinate to the others, particularly professional autonomy, patient autonomy, and consumer sovereignty' (Holsinger and Beaton 2006). These twentieth-century values may be defined thus: (1) professional autonomy: self-regulation has been the norm over the years in the healthcare community; (2) patient autonomy (respect for patients): patients expect to be provided with applicable information through verbal and/or written communication in order to be well informed concerning their health status, thus allowing informed decision-making regarding recommended treatment plans; (3) consumer sovereignty: a person's right to choose their healthcare provider and health insurance plan, which may be realigned to support a patient's right to choose a provider within a universal healthcare system; (4) patient advocacy: providers seek appropriate care for patients without regard to financial means within a system of finite resources (altruism can be considered a form of patient advocacy when healthcare providers place the interest of the patient ahead of self-interest); (5) access to care: the provision of healthcare services to individuals possessing the ability to pay for services, through third-party insurance reimbursement or governmental payments; and (6) assurance of quality of care: commitment by healthcare providers to 'best practice' care with current information through continuing education and research.

Since this twentieth-century values framework no longer appeared to meet societal needs, Priester proposed a new framework based on both essential and instrumental values. The new values framework that was proposed occurred in response to changes within society and the healthcare community. In developing the new framework, Priester (1992) determined that essential values are 'fundamental for any healthcare system: without them, a system would be deficient … instrumental values (are) primarily a means to help achieve the essential values.' The essential values include: (1) fair access: Priester places this value at the pinnacle of his twenty-first century values system, with the other four essential values strongly supporting it; (2) quality of care: 'Healthcare should maximize the likelihood of desired health outcomes for individuals and populations, and be humanely and respectfully provided' (Priester 1992); (3) efficiency: in obtaining the greatest benefit, in terms of outcomes, at the lowest cost, two important dimensions should be considered related to efficient healthcare – minimizing the costs of services offered and choosing the level, quality and make-up of services will lead to maximum excess of benefits above costs (Pauly *et al.* 1991); (4) respect for patients: patient autonomy in recent years has replaced historic medical paternalism in patient–provider relationships; (5) patient advocacy: since it is impossible for healthcare providers to serve two masters, conflicts of interest should be decided in the patient's favour.

The instrumental values that serve to support the essential values include: (1) personal responsibility: patients should be enabled to take the necessary steps to maintain and improve their health status without judgement, through patient education of risks related to unhealthy lifestyle behaviours and the offering of programmes designed to encourage good health behaviours; (2) social solidarity: a commitment to bridging gaps between dissimilar segments of the population by inclusion into the community should occur through active involvement through programmes bringing all groups of people together for the provision of healthcare services; (3) social advocacy: advancing the health status in all members of the community occurs through advocating for healthcare services for vulnerable and underserved populations while providing healthcare services for the entire population; (4) provider autonomy: healthcare providers are free to practise their profession to the best of their ability without interference and are free to accept or reject patients; (5) consumer sovereignty: patients have the freedom to choose their healthcare provider and the right to the information required to make informed personal healthcare decisions; (6) personal security: peace of mind and financial security are provided to members of the population through the provision of healthcare services that meet the health needs of the patient without resulting in financial impoverishment.

Clearly, the implementation of Priester's model would materially change the primary tenets of professionalism for the healthcare community. Priester's new values framework replaces the old professional autonomy with fair access to healthcare as the pinnacle value for healthcare providers in the twenty-first century. In his framework, four other essential values rise to importance: quality of healthcare, efficiency in its provision, respect for patients and patient advocacy. All other values play a supporting role to these key tenets of provider engagement with patients, including physician autonomy, the hallmark of twentieth-century professionalism.

Professionalism in a new century

New professional relationships

In the twenty-first century, an active dialogue has been underway to discern the significance of professionalism as a value for the healthcare professions (Leach 2004). Retaining professionalism as a core value for healthcare practitioners at both the individual and organizational levels is important since it has characterized the healthcare professions for so many years (Swick 2007). Physicians and other healthcare practitioners exhibit the attributes of professionalism on a daily basis in their practices, organizations and personal lives. This professionalism is exhibited through a variety of relationships, such as: the physician–physician relationship, resulting in respectful collaboration; the physician–patient relationship, resulting in respect and dignity, confidentiality and honesty; the physician–community relationship, resulting in social justice; the physician–healthcare system relationship, resulting in respectful interdependence; and the physician–self relationship, resulting in self-respect, self-care allowing time for renewal, and a balanced personal and professional life (ACGME 2004).

Professionalism is confirmed when patients act as advocates for their physicians and other healthcare practitioners. Patients report to each other concerning which physicians demonstrate a high level of professionalism and competence. The physician taking the time to provide high-quality care and to build a trusting relationship with a patient has taken an important step towards creating a physician advocate. The physician–patient encounter is an appropriate opportunity for physicians to demonstrate dignity and respect for patients while being actively engaged in their care. Such examples demonstrate the practice of professionalism by healthcare practitioners while engaging in patient care. Regardless of how complex the healthcare system becomes, the patient interface with healthcare practitioners will remain the prime focus of the patient's encounter with the healthcare system.

Just as twenty-first-century physicians and other healthcare practitioners differ from those of a previous century, so the typical patient has changed over the years. The twenty-first-century patient expects to play an active role in the decision-making process related to their health status. When interacting with healthcare practitioners, patients expect to receive information related to their health status and to understand the treatment options. However, the patient's desire to have a healthcare practitioner who demonstrates professionalism has not changed. In the twenty-first century, healthcare practitioner professionalism will reinforce patient expectations.

Professionalism and society

Priester (1992) addressed the significance of the community and the role it plays in healthcare. The US healthcare system has been based on the relationship of a single physician to a single patient, thus treating one at a time. The importance of caring for an entire community and considering its health status is an increasing aspect of professionalism for healthcare practitioners. The American Medical Association (AMA) *Principles of Medical Ethics* (2001) includes Section VII, 'the betterment of public health,' and Section IX, support of 'access to medical care for all people.' Social advocacy is an example of practitioners in the healthcare system engaging with those in public health to improve the overall health of a community. This concept is not new to the healthcare community but has been a part of the AMA *Principles of Medical Ethics* for many years. Section I of the *Principles of Medical Ethics* dated 7 June 1958 states, 'The principal objective of the medical profession is to render service to humanity' (American Medical Association 1958, Priester 1992). The current AMA *Principles of Medical Ethics* document states that a physician's responsibility is to the patient (first and foremost), society, colleagues and self (American Medical Association 2001). This document reflects the re-emerging value of professionalism in the medical community, indicating that the physician 'shall uphold the standards of professionalism' (American Medical Association 2001).

Societal expectations include social justice, solidarity, community awareness and the social contract. Society expects healthcare practitioners to provide a high standard of service to persons in the local community without discrimination due to race, socio-economic status or other social characteristic, promoting justice in the use of finite healthcare resources (ABIM Foundation *et al.* 2002). The social contract between healthcare practitioners and society is an important aspect of twenty-first-century professionalism. The contract is fulfilled by active participation in the local community through active involvement in professional and local organizations (Swick 2007). This level of professionalism has been questioned by some individuals and consumer interest groups who find that physician loyalty is focused on self-interest rather than on emphasizing the wellbeing of society (Humphrey 2008). However, 'civic professionalism' may be demonstrated on a societal level by physicians and other healthcare practitioners through civic engagement (Humphrey 2008).

Access to healthcare for all people regardless of ability to pay is a major issue facing healthcare systems in the twenty-first century. Professionalism in a new century requires that physicians and healthcare practitioners support this key societal demand. The American Medical Association (2001) states that an ethical physician shall 'be free to choose whom to serve,' while also supporting 'access to medical care for all people.' The highest standard of quality in medical and healthcare practice surviving the test of time will carry the healthcare professions into the twenty-first century (Swick *et al.* 2006). The ideals of the healthcare professions will be transformed in the twenty-first century through the renewal of professionalism as a value, an ever-evolving competency (Leo and Eagen 2008).

The new professionalism framework

Values provide the basis for developing a framework for the new professionalism of the twenty-first century, developed from the perspective of all four entities involved, including the healthcare provider, the individual patient, the healthcare system and society as a whole. The values that form this framework cannot be taken for granted but rather must be strived for throughout the practitioner's lifetime (Figure 11.1). The key denominator in the new professionalism framework is the healthcare practitioner who inculcates respect and dignity, commitment to excellence and accountability to the patient, the healthcare system and society. In order to practise professionalism and effectively fulfil their roles, it is imperative that healthcare practitioners maintain a balanced professional and personal life. Self-renewal of the physical (body), social (relationships with others), emotional (mind) and spiritual (spirit) dimensions in the person's life is necessary, thus intertwining the personal and professional

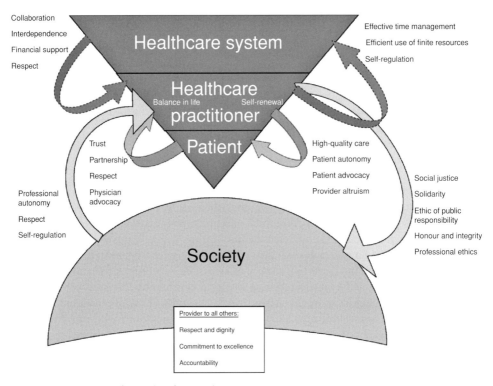

Figure 11.1 The new professionalism framework

(Covey 2004). The healthcare practitioner benefits from professional autonomy and respect from individual patients, the healthcare system and all levels of society, as well as financial support. Providing the patient with high-quality care generates practitioner advocacy, trust and respect. Additional values fulfilled by the healthcare practitioner include recognizing patient autonomy – developing a partnership with the patient in order to share necessary health status information to enable informed decision-making. A healthcare practitioner's duties extend beyond diagnosis and treatment to include altruism and patient advocacy.

Today's healthcare practitioners are an integral part of the healthcare system, which is characterized by interdependence and collaboration to provide patients with high-quality healthcare in a timely fashion. Owing to the number of patients requiring healthcare services, the practitioner needs to be well educated, practising effective time management and efficient use of finite resources.

As the twenty-first century progresses, healthcare practitioners will need to be educated and fulfil the requirements of their respective national organizations regarding licensure and certification. To benefit both society and individual patients, healthcare practitioners will practise professional autonomy as a team, supporting – versus competing with – each other. Healthcare practitioners will place an emphasis on social justice and solidarity with patients and society, and honour and integrity will be the hallmarks of the new professionalism.

References

ABIM (2001). *Project Professionalism.* www. abimfoundation.org/en/.../~/media/... /Project%20professionalism.ashx. Last accessed 20 April 2010.

ABIM Foundation, ACP-ASIM Foundation, EFIM (2002). Medical professionalism in the new millennium: a physician charter. *Annals of Internal Medicine* **136**(3), 243–246.

ABIM Foundation, ACP-ASIM Foundation, EFIM (2004). Medical professionalism in the new millennium: a physician charter. www. abimfoundation.org/professionalism/pdf_ charter/ABIM_Charter_Ins.pdf. Last accessed 13 March 2009.

ACGME (2000). *ACGME Competencies: Suggested Best Methods for Evaluation.* www. acgme.org/Outcome/assess/ToolTable.pdf. Last accessed 20 April 2010.

ACGME (2003). *ACGME General Competencies.* Accreditation Council for Graduate Medical Education. www.hmc.psu.edu/competencies/ pdfs/ACGME%20GENERAL% 20COMPETENCIES.pdf. Last accessed 29 April 2009.

ACGME (2004). *Advancing Education in Medical Professionalism. An Educational Resource from the ACGME Outcome Project Enhancing Residency Education through Outcomes Assessment.* www.acgme.org/outcome/implement/ profm_resource.pdf. Last accessed 20 April 2010.

American Medical Association (1958). *Principles of Medical Ethics.* Judicial Council: American Medical Association, 7 June. www.ama-assn. org/ama/upload/mm/369/1957_ principles.pdf. Last accessed 16 April 2010.

American Medical Association (2001). *Principles of Medical Ethics.* www.ama-assn. org/ama/pub/physician-resources/medical-ethics/ama-code-medical-ethics/principles-medical-ethics.shtml. Last accessed 17 March 2009.

Blank L, Kimball H, McDonald W, Merino J (2003). Medical professionalism in the new millennium: A physician charter 15 months later. *Annals of Internal Medicine* **138**, 839–841.

Covey S R (2004). *The 7 Habits of Highly Effective People: Restoring the Character Ethic* (rev edn). New York: Free Press.

Flexner A (1910). *Medical Education in the United States and Canada.* Boston: Merrymount Press.

Fox R C (1990). Training in caring competence in North American medicine: reforming the reforms. *Humane Medicine* **6**, 15–21.

Hafferty F W (2006). Definitions of professionalism: a search for meaning and identity. *Clinical Orthopaedics and Related Research* **449**, 193–204.

Holsinger J W, Beaton B (2006). Physician professionalism for a new century. *Clinical Anatomy* **19**, 473–479.

Humphrey H J (2008). Medical professionalism: introduction. *Perspectives in Biology and Medicine* **51**, 491–494.

Leach D C (2004). Professionalism: the formation of physicians. *American Journal of Bioethics* **4**, 11–12.

Leo T, Eagen K (2008). Professionalism education: the medical student response. *Perspectives in Biology and Medicine* **51**, 508–516.

Pauly M V, Danzon P, Feldstein P, Hoff J (1991). A plan for responsible national health insurance. *Health Affairs* **10**, 5–25.

Peabody F W (1927). The care of the patient. *Journal of the American Medical Association* **88**, 877–882.

Priester R (1992). A values framework for health system reform. *Health Affairs* **11**, 84–107.

Stevens R A (2002). Themes in the history of medical professionalism. *The Mount Sinai Journal of Medicine* **69**, 357–362.

Swick H M (1998). Academic medicine must deal with the clash of business and professional values. *Academic Medicine* **73**, 751–755.

Swick H M (2007). Viewpoint: Professionalism and humanism beyond the academic health center. *Academic Medicine* **82**, 1022–1028.

Swick H M, Bryan C S, Longo L D (2006). Beyond the physician charter: reflections on medical professionalism. *Perspectives in Biology and Medicine* **49**, 263–275.

Weiss Roberts L, Johnson M E, Brems C, Warner T D (2006). Preferences of Alaska and New Mexico psychiatrists regarding professionalism and ethics training. *Academic Psychiatry* **30**, 200–204.

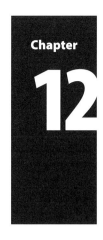
Medical professionalism in the new century

Accomplishments and challenges in the future for an American medical school

John A. Talbott

Editors' introduction

The training of professionalism in medical schools raises specific issues. Medical students may be mature, having done other things, or may come straight into medicine after finishing school. These two groups may thus have completely different views about medicine as well as professionalism. It is inevitable that personal factors will play a significant role in developing values and beliefs. Talbott, using his own experience in a medical school, illustrates the components of professionalism using the acronym HELPERS-PRO. He argues that humanism and ethics have to be subsumed under the rubric of professionalism. Humanism is at the core of the doctor–patient interaction. Altruism, autonomy, beneficence, honesty, justice, non-malfeasance and respect are the key components of medical humanism and professionalism. It is vital in the teaching and assessment of professionalism that remediation is in place. Using the notion of the disruptive physician in the hospital, Talbott notes that disrespect, hostility, swearing, lack of financial probity and conflicts of interest are some of the problems such individuals exhibit. The reasons for the increased interest in professionalism in North America are complex. The shift from utilizing histories and physical examinations to depending on high-technology diagnostic tools and the increasing numbers of persons entering the field with science rather than humanistic backgrounds is part of the issue. In addition, external factors and pressures, demands for greater accountability and productivity, restrictions placed by health maintenance organizations and increasing consumerism, together with the litigious nature of the society, have all led to increased pressures on healthcare professionals, especially doctors. In response, Talbott suggests that the definition, promotion and celebration of professionalism and the identification of deprofessionalization and remediation have to be focused on even more in the new century. Teaching ought to be multidisciplinary and timed with students' developmental levels, and better measurement of outcomes designed and implemented.

Introduction

This chapter will deal with both the accomplishments of the past and the challenges for the future that one US medical school has articulated. My goal is not to say that our way of

Professionalism in Mental Healthcare: Experts, Expertise and Expectations, ed. Dinesh Bhugra and Amit Malik. Published by Cambridge University Press. © Cambridge University Press 2011.

conceptualizing and addressing the issues is the 'correct' one but to provide one model as an example of the complex issues we have faced and will face in the future.

As disclosure, I should emphasize that while I have been in the field of psychiatry for almost half a century, I am neither trained in nor pretend to have expertise in ethics, philosophy, medical humanism or professionalism. My interest and knowledge came about more or less by chance when my then Dean (Donald E. Wilson, MD), granting me respite in 2000 after 15 years as Chair of Psychiatry, suggested I work for him to assess the state of professionalism in the medical school and propose needed changes. Thus, this is a very personal view of my journey and therefore subject to egoistic distortion.

Background

History of professionalism

Sylvia R. and Richard L. Cruess (1997a, 2000), who have been incredibly visionary pioneers in the field, trace professionalism's origins to the formation of medical guilds and universities in the Middle Ages and attribute the 'concept of the profession as a means of organizing the delivery of health services.' They state that the 'concept of professionalism came under intense scrutiny during the 1960s and 1970s (Krause 1996, Freidson 1970). The belief that physicians would be altruistic was greeted with scepticism by social scientists, and medicine was accused of putting its own welfare above that of society (Krause 1996). This occurred as the government or the private sector took control of the medical marketplace throughout the world.'

It was not only selfishness and lack of altruism that concerned the public; it was a sense that physicians had abandoned the art of medicine (which incorporated empathy, compassion, communication, manners, kindness, the ability to skilfully convey bad news, etc.) in favour of the business of medicine (Relman 1997). In preparing to write this chapter, I reviewed all the articles in the lay and scientific press that I had clipped over the past 8 years and discovered that the vast majority were news stories that tended to have similar headlines, for example, 'Doctors Urged to Mind Bedside Manners' (Adams 2005) or 'Teaching Doctors to be Nicer' (Landro 2005). A colleague of mine researching complementary medical techniques indicated that alternative medicine practitioners believe that much of their increased practice is due to physicians' insensitivity and lack of time listening to problems, what the *New York Times* (Carey 2006) headlined as 'When Trust in Doctors Erodes, Other Treatments Fill the Void'.

There were of course some blatant examples in the press of outrageous acts of unprofessionalism, such as the 'gift' of a guitar, presumed to be gratefully coercive at best and a conflict of interest at worst, by George Harrison, former member of the Beatles, to his physician when he was dying (BBC News 2004). In addition, lawyers familiar with medical malpractice felt that many such lawsuits were precipitated by patients angry about the way they were treated interpersonally more than medically.

The medical profession also heard the call for change and, by the 1990s, professional organizations – notably the ABIM (American Board of Internal Medicine) Foundation, ACP-ASIM (American College of Physicians–American Society of Internal Medicine) Foundation and the European Federation of Internal Medicine (American Board of Internal Medicine 1995, ABIM Foundation *et al.* 2002, ABIM Foundation *et al.* 2003); regulatory bodies, through disciplinary actions (Papadakis *et al.* 2004); and faculty, students and graduates – became concerned with identifying unprofessional behaviour and remedying it.

The ABIM Foundation *et al.* (2002) issued reports and a Charter on Professionalism that essentially defined what medical professionals and the field needed to focus on. This Charter called for the:

Principle of primacy of patient welfare
Principle of patient autonomy
Principle of social justice
Commitment to professional competence
Commitment to honesty with patients
Commitment to patient confidentiality
Commitment to maintaining appropriate relations with patients
Commitment to improving quality of care
Commitment to improving access to care
Commitment to a just distribution of finite resources
Commitment to scientific knowledge
Commitment to maintaining trust by managing conflicts of interest
Commitment to professional responsibilities.

The Project and the Charter drew heavily upon the work of Swick (2000), who said a definition of 'Medical professionalism, then, comprises the following set of behaviors, physicians

subordinate their own interests to the interests of others,
adhere to high ethical and moral standards,
respond to societal needs, and their behaviors reflect a social contract with the communities served,
evince core humanistic values, including honesty and integrity, caring and compassion, altruism and empathy, respect for others, and trustworthiness,
exercise accountability for themselves and for their colleagues,
demonstrate a continuing commitment to excellence,
exhibit a commitment to scholarship and to advancing their field,
deal with high levels of complexity and uncertainty,
reflect upon their actions and decisions.'

At the University of Maryland School of Medicine, we tried in 2000 to encompass all of these in an acronym that would convey their essence. What we came up with was **HELPERS-PRO**, standing for:

Humanism
Ethics
Lifelong learning
Physicians subordinating themselves to their patients
Ethical behaviour
Research subjects
Sensitivity to age, culture, disability, diversity and gender
Professionalism
Respect for patients, families and colleagues
Other (death and dying, impairment, sexual and aggressive behaviour, physician–industry relationships).

Professionalism and/or versus humanism?

The acronym that we used for professionalism subsumed humanism (as well as ethics) under professionalism, which deserves some comment. As a continent in which we have 141 medical schools in 50 states and 13 provinces and territories (I include Canada here because so much seminal work has come from our northern neighbours), it is expectable that different schools call their umbrella concept different things. I think the term that serves as the umbrella under which everything else is incorporated is less important than the fact that projects and efforts incorporate all of Swick's items.

But medical humanism has its own historical background in the United States. According to their website, Humanism in Medicine, 'Arnold and Sandra Gold and a dedicated group of Columbia colleagues, medical educators and community leaders began the [Arnold P. Gold, M.D.] Foundation in the fall of 1988 with the power of an idea – to nurture and preserve the tradition of the caring physician.'

In 1989, the University of Chicago's Pritzker School of Medicine held its first white coat ceremony to 'mark the transition between the initial science course curriculum and the beginning of their clinical and direct patient care training' (20th Anniversary). Subsequently, it has been adopted in almost every medical school on the continent to mark a transition and assumption of the role of a humanistic physician, and instrumental to this phenomenon has been the tireless work and support of Arnold P. Gold, MD and Sandra O. Gold, EdD.

The Foundation has been a force behind other humanism activities. In 1991, the first of a national series of 'Commencement Awards' were initiated at Columbia University College of Physicians & Surgeons to recognize exemplary role models and entailed presenting an award for a faculty member and graduating medical student. In addition, the Foundation provided grants:

- To promote another ceremony called the 'Student Clinician Ceremony' to mark the transition between the preclinical and clinical years
- To initiate the Gold Humanism Honor Society, honouring approximately 10% of the graduating class at the end of medical school, which now has chapters in over 80 medical schools
- For innovative programmes
- For programmes and lectureships at the American Association of Medical Colleges
- For the distribution of films and books on medical humanism.

The cumulative effect of these ceremonies, awards and honours cannot be underestimated. They initiate, reinforce and reward humanistic medical practice and are visible reminders to faculty, staff and students of the importance we all place on humanistic medicine.

Philosophy and ethics

While the history of philosophic and ethical principles predates Hippocrates, these principles remain important underpinnings of our programmes in professionalism and humanism. Bookshelves of books and texts have been devoted to these subjects, and so I will not attempt to detail them; however, running parallel to the historical development of medical humanism and professionalism are such areas as:

Altruism
Autonomy

Beneficence

Honesty

Justice

Non-malfeasance, and

Respect.

Oaths

An important way to institutionalize and highlight the values and goals of professionalism and humanism is through the use of Oaths, Codes and Charters. Modern iterations of these are all derivative in some sense of the Oath of Hippocrates (460–370 BC) and Oath and Code of Maimonides (1135–1204). So many medical schools have various codes and oaths that it would be difficult to list them, but a Google search or look at a sample website ('university') reveals the scope and details intended to be emphasized. The most contemporary one is the aforementioned Charter on Professionalism (ABIM Foundation *et al.* 2002).

What have we learnt over the past few decades?

An example of the sort of programme in an individual medical school that seeks to be comprehensive in promoting professionalism and humanism is at the University of Maryland. In 2000, the Dean asked me to undertake an examination of the undergraduate programme, from the admissions process to the graduation requirements, and come up with recommendations to improve the situation, which he deemed in need of improvement. My report, *Becoming a Physician at the University of Maryland School of Medicine (Becoming a Physician: Helpers-Pro)*, contained 31 recommendations that he approved immediately and for which he authorized implementation (Talbott 2001).

Admissions process

At the front end, we wished to improve the professionalism of students admitted to the school and added questions to the admissions interviews that better plumbed these issues, such as:

1. What are the values and ethical principles that have guided you through life?
2. Discuss a situation in which your values were challenged and how you dealt with it?
3. How do you see the profession of medicine as different from other professions?
4. Describe a situation in which you put someone else's needs before your own.
5. Describe a situation where it was a challenge for you to behave 'professionally'.
6. How do you handle competing demands on your time?
7. Do you think a physician's attire/appearance influences the doctor–patient relationship?
8. Give an example of what you would consider to be unprofessional behaviour in a medical student.
9. What would you do if you observed another student cheating?
10. Give an example of what you would consider to be unprofessional behaviour in a physician.
11. To what extent should an individual sacrifice himself/herself to fulfil a job? What are your criteria for a fulfilling career?

Identification and remediation of unprofessional student behaviour

An area that has really been pioneered is the identification of unprofessional behaviour. Almost all medical schools have designed instruments and methods to assess such problems, exemplary models of which were developed at the University of Toronto (Task Force 2001) and the University of Michigan (David Stern 2006).

At the instigation of the faculty, particularly those in the basic sciences who felt that they could identify unprofessional behaviour in the first days of medical school and the clinical faculty, who opined that we must be able to remedy unprofessional behaviour before students entered their third-year clinical clerkships, we implemented an evaluation (Talbott 2005) of each student in each course as well as in each clinical rotation (adapting instruments designed at the University of Toronto).

After a year, we superseded this rather clumsy and time-consuming process with an expansion of our Academic Advancement Committee's mission to include professional as well as academic assessments of each student after each course or rotation, since the committee consisted of all course and clerkship directors. These bi-yearly reviews are of great help when it comes to answering the questions about professionalism on the Medical Student Performance Evaluation (MSPE), formerly known as the 'Dean's letter', as well as for nominations to the Gold Humanism Honor Society.

In some cases, such as lying, writing fraudulent records, etc., the student is recommended for either dismissal or referral to the school's Judicial Board at the time of the initial discussion. Obviously, there are also even rarer incidences when the misconduct is so serious, e.g. a criminal act, that immediate assessment and action are taken before the monthly meeting of the Advancement Committee.

Because students indicated that they wished to have a bigger role in identification, peer assistance and teaching about professionalism, we instituted an anonymous student–student reporting system (which had to be abandoned after 3 years of success due to a system-wide computer 'upgrade'), a 'suggestion/criticism box' on the student intranet/website (based on that from the University of Virginia called 'The Listening Post') and a Student Advisory Committee to the Project Director that took over parts of the orientations on professionalism as well as special projects and papers.

David Stern (personal communication, 2003) at the University of Michigan looked at all the data in students' admissions folders and found that soft signs of poor citizenship, such as not completing training modules or filling out forms, predicted later problems with professionalism. We found that multiple requests for postponement of examinations during medical school predicted later considerations of remediation or dismissal. And Maxine Papadakis *et al.* at the University of California (2004) found that unprofessional acts in medical school predicted later disciplinary actions by licensing boards. Thus, we take any repeated violation of professional behaviour extremely seriously since it is obvious that behaviour recurs unless remediated.

Remediation of professionalism difficulties occurs in multiple forms, including meetings with the deans of student affairs, director of the Professionalism Project, mentoring and closer supervision, counselling or psychiatric treatment and individual projects such as writing papers on issues of professionalism. Often, a single, simple meeting with someone in authority is all it takes; more often, the process involves multiple meetings after separate incidents over a period of a month, but rarely is it necessary to have students repeat rotations and, even more rarely, undergo dismissal.

Teaching professionalism

In addition, we have learnt a great deal about teaching professionalism. Spurred again by Richard and Sylvia Cruess (1997b), most medical schools in North America have entered this area, one in which there was no attention a few years ago. There are still contrarians who believe we cannot teach the subject, only choose students best suited for professional careers, and not all subjects have been successfully tackled – but progress is there. (See Chapter 8 for potential methods in teaching.)

We began to improve professionalism through a total revamping of orientations and the reworking of a course called 'Introduction to Clinical Medicine', where problem-based learning, history taking, physical diagnosis and Observed Standardized Clinical Examinations (OSCEs) were augmented with attention to the following: medical ethics and ethical behaviour; death and dying, pain and palliation, breaking bad news; house staff treatment of students; communication, the doctor–patient relationship, boundaries; strains and stresses of becoming and being a physician (e.g. substance abuse, divorce); religion and spirituality; cultural, ethnic, gender, sexual and socio-economic diversity; patient safety/medical errors; physician–industry relationships and gifts from industry; impairment; treating the VIP, HIV patients, smokers, the mentally and physically handicapped; and sexual harassment (Talbott 2006).

Faculty and house staff development

Finally, faculty development is an area of concern. We have become aware that the behaviour of the faculty and house staff far outweighs what we say, and experts such as Frederic Hafferty (1995) have emphasized the power of the 'hidden curriculum'. But it goes beyond that; teachers are not adequately rewarded for teaching, teachers are not taught how to teach and teaching professionalism and humanism is not for everyone. This is an area where we at the University of Maryland lag far behind other institutions that have implemented vigorous programmes to improve teaching and faculty professionalism. A major problem is that the primary role models for students are house officers, who in the United States are paid by and are responsible to the academic hospitals and their clinical departments and are thus only indirectly influenceable by our programmes.

The 'disruptive physician' in the hospital

Parallel to the focus those in medical education have placed on professionalism and unprofessional behaviour is concern on the part of hospitals with what has come to be known as the 'disruptive physician'. While medical educators have focused on items such as altruism, responsibility to the patient and death and dying, hospital administrators are rightly concerned with medical errors, dysfunctional teams and disrespect in the workplace.

Most of the early literature on the subject was in medical administration publications (such as that by Rosenstein *et al.* 2002) and documents the personal and economic toll of misbehaviour, but more recently scientific publications have published studies (such as by Bohigian *et al.* 2005) and editorials. The concern has reached the level of the US quasi-regulatory body, the Joint Commission on the Accreditation of Health Care Organizations (JCAHO), which has issued a policy on the identification and remediation of such behaviour (O'Reilly 2008).

Because of opposition from the American Medical Association, implementation of this policy has been postponed a year. However, individual hospitals, such as my own, had already put in place a process of defining, identifying and remediating such behaviour.

In 2003, the medical staff leadership at the University of Maryland Medical Center appointed a task force to draw up a Code of Professional Conduct. It surveyed codes throughout the country and, after considerable discussion and some revision, adopted that in use at the Dartmouth/Hitchcock Medical Center in New Hampshire. The areas covered included respect for persons, patient confidentiality, personal ethics and property and laws, honesty, integrity and responsibility for patient care, awareness of limitations, professional growth and lifelong learning, deportment as a professional, responsibility for peer behaviour, avoiding conflicts of interest and integrity in research.

Each attending physician signs the Code upon being hired and credentialed and then yearly afterwards when he or she is re-credentialed. After the Code was approved and promulgated, a committee was appointed to screen complaints of violations in the Code and remedy the situation. In the 5 years since the Code was implemented, 50 complaints have been received (amounting to about one a month) that concerned 33 persons, 21 of whom belonged to the Departments of Surgery or Anesthesia.

The results are as follows (Talbott 2008): all except four were complaints about physicians, half of the complaints were from nurses but four were from physicians, and all were for disrespect, yelling, harassment, humiliation, verbal attacks, condescension, rudeness, hostility and swearing, except one about alleged financial chicanery with drug company monies and another about a request for sex that was demeaning and mocking.

In all cases, the committee seeks to hear from both sides as well as from observers and supervisors. The best resolutions are when the remedy sought by the person making the complaint, usually a simple face-to-face apology, is carried out with sincerity. In the worst case, the committee advised the chief medical officer of the hospital (who sits *ex officio* on the committee) to subsidize an intervention by an outside consulting firm on an entire division. In many cases, we have heard that chiefs of service themselves intervene before misbehaviour is reported, telling physicians that 'you don't want to be hauled before that committee.'

Exemplary behaviour

Unfortunately, much of our time was and is spent on misbehaviour and much too little on exemplary behaviour. However, there are opportunities to acknowledge such exemplars. For instance, we received the following nomination for a student to the Gold Humanism Honor Society:

Ms. X is the epitome of professionalism and ethics in a medical student, and is the type of individual that the UMB School of Medicine strives to cultivate as a future physician. I have personally witnessed countless instances of her example of integrity, morals, and respect for others, throughout the first 3 years of medical school. This sentiment is echoed by many of my fellow classmates, residents, and attending physicians, who have mentioned her professionalism and integrity several months after completing a rotation with her. To receive these sort of remarks well after the fact means that she has made a lasting impression in her profession and has achieved something very special in her personal encounters with others. Of utmost importance to her, however, is that she holds her patients in the highest regard, and displays an unwavering compassion, altruism, and empathy in her care of them. She also demonstrates a continuing commitment to excellence and exhibits a commitment to scholarship that is unrivaled amongst our fellow classmates. She is an inspiration to her fellow students, the physicians she works under, and especially to her patients.

This sort of report not only raises the likelihood that she will be among the 10 to 15% of the graduating class selected to the Honor Society, but its inclusion in the 'Dean's letter' that goes to the Residency Directors to whose programmes she is applying will enhance her application.

In addition, four student members of the Society also receive named awards at graduation (that carry stipends with them), and all members select six house officers and one faculty member to also be honoured during graduation week. Without doubt more needs to be done, and we are considering the suggestion of implementing a Web-based red rose (or other positive symbol) award, which would be given immediately after a good deed or teaching moment.

Internet presence

It should be noted that one way we have tried to make this a comprehensive programme is to have all the information about it on a single website. Examples of the links to various aspects of the programme follow:

- The Professionalism website
    - http://medschool.umaryland.edu/Professionalism/default.asp

- The Evaluation page
    - http://medschool.umaryland.edu/Professionalism/Evaluation.asp

- The Humanism page
    - http://medschool.umaryland.edu/Professionalism/Humanism/default.asp

- The Feedback loop
    - http://medschool.umaryland.edu/professionalism/feedback

- Gifts from industry
    - http://medschool.umaryland.edu/professionalism/gifts.asp

- Oaths and Codes
    - http://medschool.umaryland.edu/professionalism/Oaths.asp

How the US healthcare system and threats are changing professionalism

As the only developed country in the world (except for South Africa) that does not have a national health programme, the United States has somewhat different problems that affect physicians than the rest of the world. For example, because not all Americans have health insurance, physicians spend inordinate amounts of time justifying unreimbursed care. And even if patients have insurance, physicians spend inordinate amounts of time filling out paperwork, billing and collecting fees and dealing with governmental and private insurers.

Rosenstein *et al.* (2002) cited 'external pressures' that physicians feel cause them to be 'demoralized and harbor a victim mentality':

Lower compensation

Demands for greater accountability and productivity

Governmental oversight

Managed care restrictions

Consumerism

Increasing liability risks.

At the time this chapter was edited, the results of the legislation that President Obama signed into law to reform healthcare in the United States are unknown, and whether this plan will reduce or aggravate the current feeling of demoralization and victim mentality is equally unclear. The following anecdote may illustrate the perception of lapses in professionalism not being the physician's responsibility but a consequence of outside forces.

The author, in his role as chair of the Code of Professional Conduct process, is often asked to give talks and Grand Rounds by various departments and divisions. After one such session, a physician whom a nurse had complained about complained himself that the author could not possibly understand how much stress he was under, to which he replied that in a year observing combat physicians in Vietnam, always under the threat of fire, he had not seen or heard of one incident of unprofessional behaviour. (This complainer has not had any subsequent complaints made about him.)

Professionalism in the new century

It is always a risky business predicting the future. As I have pointed out elsewhere, who would have predicted the fall of the Berlin Wall, the collapse of the global economy or the election of an African-American President of the United States, where visible racism still exists.

However, I think some things are on the table for action:

1. Weaving all the elements together in a whole cloth. A major task facing us is to put together all we know about professionalism (its definition, promotion, celebration, teaching and dissemination) and unprofessionalism (its definition, identification, evaluation, quantification, remediation and follow-up) into a comprehensive programme that all involved will embrace together.
2. Teaching and training in interdisciplinary groups and among clinical teams so that respect and equal value are placed on all activities and involvements.
3. Measuring the outcomes of our efforts. At present, we have but crude instruments to measure with – exit interviews, complaint files, staff turnover rates, dismissal or remediation actions and surveys of staff satisfaction/dissatisfaction.
4. Better melding of university educational and hospital clinical efforts so that even in the absence of joint governance, everyone entering the enterprise appreciates the goal of achieving more professionalism, whether in educational, research, administration, community or clinical activities.
5. Teaching and training all involved about all the elements necessary to achieve the most professional result when such training is applicable to the developmental process. It is premature to teach about death or dying or research ethics 3 years before students need to know such material, just as it is too late to learn how to talk about difficult subjects 2 years after entering patient settings. Ethics is a perfect example of a field of knowledge that needs to be tailor-made to the stage of development the learner is at.

6. Teaching subjects we are not terribly comfortable about teaching, such as spirituality and religion, cultural differences, comportment and deportment, listening, self-reflection, civility and compassion, as well as implementing new activities, such as service learning.
7. Utilizing the Internet and other electronic means to improve communication, professionalism and humanism rather than distance ourselves from colleagues, staffs and patients.
8. Communicating among ourselves so that individuals beginning projects or efforts stand on the shoulders of others rather than reinvent wheels.
9. Leverage the power of support from above (i.e. the Dean and CEO) as well as the involvement of those in learning situations (i.e. students and house officers) in the pursuit of professionalism.
10. Finishing the task of eliminating conflicts of interest involving industry, especially the drug industry.

Summary

Medical professionalism in North America has been a work in progress for many years. While the concepts of guilds and professions go back hundreds of years, it was really only with the introduction of the white coat ceremony at the University of Chicago in 1989, the subsequent attention on medical humanism on the parts of Sandra and Arnold Gold in New York City and the focus on professionalism by the ABIM Foundation *et al.* that medical schools in the United States and Canada began to focus on medical professionalism and medical humanism.

Much has happened in the two decades since then, and this chapter has summarized the achievements and knowledge about professionalism, the changes and threats, past and present, to our profession and the challenges that face us in the future.

References

20th Anniversary of the White Coat Ceremony. www.articlesbase.com/clothing-articles/20th-anniversary-of-the-white-coat-ceremony-819135.html. Last accessed 1 April 2009.

ABIM Foundation, ACP-ASIM Foundation, EFIM (2002). Medical professionalism in the new millennium: a physician charter. *Annals of Internal Medicine* **136**(3), 243–246.

ABIM Foundation, ACP-ASIM Foundation, EFIM (2003). Medical professionalism in the new millennium: a physician charter 15 months later. Letters to the Editor and Editorial. *Annals of Internal Medicine* **138**(10), 839–841, 844–846, 851–855.

Adams D (21 March 2005). Doctors urged to mind bedside manners. *American Medical News* **48**(11), 1.

American Board of Internal Medicine (1995). *Project Professionalism*. www.abim.org/pdf/publications/professionalism.pdf. Last accessed 1 April 2009.

BBC News (17 January 2004). Beatle's guitar lawsuit settled. http://news.bbc.co.uk/2/hi/entertainment/3405567.stm. Last accessed 15 January 2009.

Bohigian G M, Bondurant R, Croughan J (2005). The impaired and disruptive physician: the Missouri Physicians' Health Program–an update (1995–2002). *Journal of Addictive Diseases* **24**(1), 13–23.

Carey B (3 February 2006). When trust in doctors erodes, other treatments fill the void. *New York Times* p. 1.

Cruess R, Cruess S (1997a). Teaching medicine as a profession in the service of healing. *Academic Medicine* **72**(1), 941–952.

Cruess S, Cruess R (1997b). Teaching professionalism. *British Medical Journal* **314**, 1674–1677.

Cruess S R, Cruess R L (2000). Professionalism: a contract between medicine and society. *Canadian Medical Association Journal* **162**(5), 673–675.

Freidson E (1970). *Professional Dominance: The Social Structure of Medical Care*. Chicago: Aldine.

Hafferty F W (1995). Assessing the impact of the hidden curriculum on the process and content of medical education. *Academic Medicine* **71**(6), 629–630.

Humanism in Medicine. http://humanism-in-medicine.org/. Last accessed 1 April 2009.

Krause E A (1996). *Death of the Guilds: Professions, States, and the Advance of Capitalism, 1930 to the Present*. New Haven: Yale University Press.

Landro L (28 September 2005). Teaching doctors to be nicer. *Wall Street Journal*, p. D1.

O'Reilly K B (18 August 2008). New Joint Commission standard tells hospitals to squelch disruptive behaviors: doctors worry about the new requirement, saying hospitals could misuse bad – behavior policies. *American Medical News*, p. 1.

Papadakis M A, Hodgson C S, Teherani A, Kohatsu N D (2004). Unprofessional behavior in medical school is associated with subsequent disciplinary action by a state medical board. *Academic Medicine* **79**(3), 244–249.

Relman A (1997). Medicine: business or art. *P&S Journal*, **17**(3). http://cumc.columbia.edu/news/journal/journal-o/archives/jour_v17n03_0027.html. Last accessed 25 April 2010.

Rosenstein A H, Russell H, Lauve R (2002). Disruptive physician behavior contributes to nursing shortage. *Physician Executive* **28**(6), 8–11.

Stern D T (2006). *Measuring Medical Professionalism*. New York: Oxford University Press.

Swick H M (2000). Toward a normative definition of medical professionalism. *Academic Medicine* **75**(6), 612–616.

Talbott J A (2001). *Becoming a Physician at the University of Maryland School of Medicine (Becoming a Physician: Helpers-Pro)*. http://medschool.umaryland.edu/Professionalism/Report.asp. Last accessed 16 January 2009.

Talbott J A (2005). Professionalism: its definition, evaluation and teaching in medical school. *Journal of Veterinary Medicine* **32**(2), 237–241.

Talbott J A (2006). Professionalism: why now, what is it, how do we do something? *Journal of Cancer Education* **21**(3), 118–122.

Talbott J A (2008). A Code of Professional Conduct: Does It Really Work? RIME poster presented at the 2008 Annual Meeting of the American Association of Medical Colleges, San Antonio, TX, 2–4 November 2008.

Task Force on Professionalism in Undergraduate Medicine at the University of Toronto (May 2001).

University of Maryland School of Medicine HELPERS-PRO website. http://medschool. umaryland.edu/Professionalism/Oaths.asp. Last accessed 16 January 2009.

University of Virginia. *The Listening Post.* www.med – ed.Virginia.edu/listen/. Last accessed 9 April 2009.

13

Ethical foundations of professionalism

James E. Sabin and H. Steven Moffic

Editors' introduction

Professional practice, irrespective of the field, has to be ethical. As our knowledge, views and beliefs about ethical practice change in response to external and internal factors, it is inevitable that the profession will respond accordingly and, if required, change the practice and components of professionalism. It is essential that these changes do not occur in a vacuum without any consultation with stakeholders. Sabin and Moffic note that often there is no or limited discussion of ethical values in the profession. They emphasize the point using the US example where an external pressure on beds and a demand to discharge seriously mentally ill individuals sooner raises an ethical dilemma for the professionals. Religious values may offer one source of professional ethics, but professionals should not be openly proselytizing about their own personal religious values and beliefs. Whilst discussing religion, Sabin and Moffic point out that the Hippocratic Oath is sworn to pagan gods, and its most extensive topic (duties owed to one's teachers) is associated with values attributed to ancient guilds. They also raise questions as to why the Oath remains so important two and a half millennia later, although efforts have been made to modernize it. The ethics of healthcare professions should result from the ethics and experience of providing and receiving healthcare itself. The illness, healthcare and the act of profession provide the core of ethical values and norms. The social contract approach differs and encourages ethics related to stakeholders as well. These authors argue that a reductionist approach and mind–body dualism lead to a very mechanistic approach to doctor–patient interaction. Ethics are also related to professions, organizations and society. Therefore, clinicians have to walk a tightrope in balancing broader and often competing demands. Sabin and Moffic argue that ethics must go beyond being platitudes or powerless ideals. A major challenge within the profession is to maintain a holistic ethical perspective within healthcare delivery.

Introduction

Ethics is central to what makes medicine a profession.[1] Society confers an honoured status and the privilege of self-regulation on medicine only to the degree to which it

---

[1] We recognize that psychiatry is only one among several mental health professions and that 'mental health' is broader than 'psychiatry'. However, as the historical literature on health professional ethics has largely focused on medicine, we frequently use the terms 'medicine', 'psychiatry' and 'medical ethics'. These and similar locutions should be seen as referring to the wider domains of

Professionalism in Mental Healthcare: Experts, Expertise and Expectations, ed. Dinesh Bhugra and Amit Malik. Published by Cambridge University Press. © Cambridge University Press 2011.

believes that physicians possess distinctive skill at healing and embody a uniquely altruistic ethical orientation. Without societal recognition for skill at healing and fidelity to an ethic of altruism, medicine would continue to be a *job*, but its status as a *profession* would disappear.

In the United States, a famous ruling in 1928 by Justice Benjamin Cardozo, later on the Supreme Court, is often cited to convey society's vision of the duty of trust held by a profession dedicated to the wellbeing of those it serves:

Many forms of conduct permissible in a workaday world for those acting at arm's length, are forbidden to those bound by fiduciary ties. A trustee is held to something stricter than the morals of the market place. Not honesty alone, but the punctilio of an honor the most sensitive, is then the standard of behavior. As to this there has developed a tradition that is unbending and inveterate. (New York Court of Appeals 1928)

In most societies students take an oath at the point of transition from apprentice-in-training to physician. This historical ritual shows just how central ethics is to what makes medicine a profession and not simply a job. In taking the oath, newly recognized physicians make a solemn pledge to conduct themselves in accord with a tradition sanctified by God or some other deeply respected source of morality. The point is not that every graduate is contemplating the moral significance of the pledge they are making. Many, perhaps most, have more mundane things in mind! But the ritual signifies that the medical profession and the societies within which the profession exists believe that students *should* be making a serious moral commitment at the point at which they enter the ranks of physicians (Sulmasy 1999).

In our experience, we mental health professionals rarely discuss or even think about the ultimate ethical foundations of our profession in the course of our everyday work. Seeking to help people recover from mental disorders seems so obviously to be a good thing that in ordinary circumstances we feel no need to ask, 'what makes this work so important?' But in unsettled circumstances, as at present when hospitals are discharging patients 'sicker and quicker', community programmes and psychotherapy are often poorly funded, and many psychiatrists find themselves pigeonholed into the narrow role of 'medication manager', asking what values we stand for can be important practically as well as theoretically. A clear understanding of the foundations of professional ethics can help individual mental health clinicians to evaluate and respond to their professional circumstances and the profession itself in its dealings with society.

If ethics is so central to medical and psychiatric professionalism, where does it come from and what is its specific content? In our view, professional ethics can be derived from three *sources*: from *outside* healthcare, especially through religious perspectives on human needs; from *within* healthcare, through analysis of the existential structure of the care relationship itself; and *between* the health professions and wider society, through the social contract between society and the medical profession. In terms of the *content* of professional ethics, we regard the pronouncements of professional societies and other health organizations as efforts to specify the essential components of professional commitments. From among the multitude of codes we use the Physician Charter as our example.

'mental health' and 'health professional ethics'. Similarly, we recognize that some mental health professionals prefer 'client' to 'patient' and that some recipients of treatment prefer 'consumer' or, among US activists, 'survivor', but for grammatical simplicity we use 'patient' throughout.

Religion as a source of professional ethics

Historically, there has been substantial overlap between religion and what the modern world thinks of as healthcare. In the Christian tradition there was no dichotomy between Jesus as prophet/teacher and Jesus as healer. In Buddhist tradition monks provided medical and nursing care as well as spiritual guidance. In Jewish tradition the Oath of Maimonides, a physician and rabbi, is widely recognized. And even today many Hindus do a puja to the gods before consulting a health professional. Most religions recognize how much modern medicine has to offer but hold that God determines how earthly life unfolds, as in the aphorism 'man proposes; God disposes!'

Religious *theologies* put forward views of the ultimate nature of being – how the universe came to be and the role of humans in it. Religious *ethics* put forward views about the rights and wrongs of human conduct. Religious health professionals can derive a broad professional ethic from their understanding of the sacred and the requirements for right conduct that their faith teaches.

Christianity, Islam and Judaism, as monotheistic religions, teach that humanity is God's creation. Human life is seen as sacred because humans participate in or reflect God's holiness. Caring for one's own health shows respect for God's handiwork. Failing to care for oneself – the extreme form of which is suicide – is an affront to God. And for all major religions, providing care for those who are vulnerable and in need, whether from poverty or illness, is a central commitment. For the faithful, health professionals are literally carrying out God's work.

Unlike the monotheistic religions and Hinduism, with its pantheon of multiple gods, Buddhism does not posit a Supreme Being or creator god. The Four Noble Truths identify the source of human suffering as craving and ignorance and the goal for human perfection as Nirvana. The Eightfold Path prescribes a programme of right conduct. In the Buddhist view, all people, including health professionals, should follow this ethical code (Keown 2004):

Medical ethics in Buddhism involves essentially the application of the wider principles of religious ethics to problems in a more specialized field … What is to be done and not to be done by the physician will be determined by the same moral principles which determine what is to be done and not to be done by a monk … (p. 178)

Several of the terms health professionals use to describe the personal meaning we derive from our roles in healthcare have religious roots. 'Calling', now defined 'an occupation, profession, or career' (Heritage Dictionary 1979), originally referred to a call that came directly from God. 'Mission', in the sense of 'a self-imposed duty', originally meant foreign travel to spread the word of God. 'Vocation', whose first definition is now secular – 'a regular occupation or profession'; especially, one 'for which one is specially suited or qualified' – originally signified a call from God to enter religious life. And even for non-believers, the clinical encounter may be experienced as a 'sacred space'. Thus, for atheists as well as clinicians of faith, the moral seriousness of the major religions – and the way that religions engage with questions about the meaning of life, suffering and death – inform approaches to the ethics of professionalism (Sulmasy 2009).

It is not immediately obvious why the Hippocratic Oath, whose pledge is sworn to pagan gods and whose most extensive topic (duties owed to one's teachers) involves the concerns of an ancient guild, is cited so frequently and with such reverence today. In our view there are four main reasons for its durability. First, the Oath forcefully specifies healing and the avoidance of harm as the primary aims for medicine: 'Into whatever homes I go, I will enter them for the benefit of the sick, avoiding any voluntary act of impropriety or corruption...and I will do no harm or injustice to them.' Second, it emphasizes the importance of confidentiality: 'Whatever I see or hear in the lives of my patients, whether in connection with my professional practice or not, which ought not to be spoken of outside, I will keep secret, as considering all such things to be private.' Third, it evokes a sense of deep moral commitment: 'In purity and according to divine law will I carry out my life and my art.' Finally, and perhaps most importantly, it connects the contemporary physician to a noble 2500-year-old moral community: 'So long as I maintain this Oath faithfully and without corruption, may it be granted to me to partake of life fully and the practice of my art, gaining the respect of all men for all time.' The distinctive strength of the Oath is the broad moral vision it provides of medical care as a sacred calling. It is not a theology for modern physicians, but it is like a religious document in deriving from biblical times and its multiple invocations of holiness.

Existential factors as a source of professional ethics

Edmund Pellegrino is the leading example of the effort to derive professional ethics from within medicine itself through analysis of the existential structure of clinical practice (Pellegrino 2006). Although some philosophers contest the possibility of doing this (Veatch 2001), Pellegrino believes that if we understand what the doctor–patient relationship is *for* and the virtues that accomplishing its purposes require, we can derive a strong, persuasive, non-relativistic foundation for professional ethics. Because it is grounded in clinical experience, the existential approach is likely to have strong face validity for mental health clinicians.

In Pellegrino's view, the ethics of the healing professions can, and should, be derived from the experience of providing and receiving healthcare itself. He argues that three phenomena – the fact of illness, the act of profession and the process of care – if understood properly, provide a coherent basis for professional ethics.

Pellegrino draws his description of 'the fact of illness' from acute medical situations:

>...some of the things we associate most closely with being human involve the capacity to use our bodies for trans-bodily and outwardly directed purposes. In a state of illness the body is no longer our ready instrument; it becomes, instead, the center of our concern. It begins to tyrannize, to make demands; it has to be listened to, taken somewhere for help. In a sense, there's a split between the self and the body: one steps back, as it were, and begins to look at one's body; the unity of body and self that had previously existed is fractured somewhat...The fragility of our human existence comes before us bluntly when we experience illness. We have, therefore, in the fact of illness, a wounded state of humanity. (p. 67)

Mental health clinicians will rightly see Pellegrino's focus on the body alone as the source of the 'wounded state' of illness too limited. While the ailments we see in mental health practice always involve the body (without a functioning brain, psychiatric ailments would not exist), psychiatric conditions are more likely to alienate us from our 'self' than from our 'body'. But Pellegrino's argument can easily be extended to recognize the fact that psychiatric conditions cause their own forms of suffering, dysfunction and 'woundedness'. The reality of suffering and dysfunction is the starting place for existential professional ethics.

Pellegrino similarly describes 'the act of profession' in terms of acute medicine, technical interventions and vulnerable patients who have limited understanding of their condition:

The relationship between someone who is ill and someone who promises to help is perforce a relationship of inequality…The physician-patient healing relationship is of its nature an unequal relationship built on vulnerability and on a promise. (p. 67)

But even for knowledgeable patients who are being treated with psychotherapy – the most collaborative and least 'unequal' of all treatments – there is an asymmetry in that clinicians make an explicit (or implicit) promise to use their skills to serve the patient and help to restore health and wellbeing to the extent that current knowledge allows. The prototypical clinical dyad involves a patient who experiences distress and a clinician who promises a good faith effort to help.

Pellegrino identifies the third pillar of professional ethics with 'the act of medicine' – the skilful application of current knowledge to promote healing. Praiseworthy healing efforts must be 'medically competent', but technical competence is not all that is required:

A good decision will fit this particular person, at this age and situation in life, with this person's aspirations, expectations, and values…it is in the relationships involved in the triad of the fact of illness, the fact of profession, and the act of medicine that the obligations of the physician and the patient to each other are born. (pp. 67–68)

This kind of fine-grained attention to the individual patient as a psychological being and to the nuances of the clinical relationship is the hallmark of mental health practice. Contemporary mental health practice makes the requirement that treatment 'fit this particular person', a core expectation for competent care. And as collaborators with colleagues in other specialties, mental health clinicians often play an important role in elucidating a patient's 'aspirations, expectations and values.'

The existential approach to professional ethics concludes that if we contemplate the encounter between a vulnerable patient and a health professional who promises to offer the potential for healing, the content of professional ethics and the virtues of the ethical clinician become obvious, especially: *trustworthiness* (since care is based on a promise); *benevolence* (since the promise is to help and to prevent avoidable harms); *intellectual honesty* (since clarity about our own capacities and the areas where we need the help of others is crucial to avoiding harm); *compassion* (since entering our patients' situations and feeling something of their plight is necessary to attune treatment to the individual); and *truthfulness* (since patients are owed the knowledge that allows them to make informed choices) (Pellegrino and Thomasma 1993).

Clinicians of faith who derive their understanding of professional ethics from their religious beliefs may see the effort to base professionalism on the internal structure of healthcare as too superficial to provide a secure ethical foundation. At the other extreme, clinicians who understand professional ethics in terms of a social contract between medicine and its external stakeholders may see the existential effort as presumptuous, 'playing God' by unilaterally decreeing to others how the ethics of the health professions should be understood. But in our view the existential approach makes a distinctively valuable contribution through its intense focus on the deep moral commitment we clinicians make to our patients when we undertake treatment.

Social contract as a source of professional ethics

The religious and existential sources of professional ethics are relatively timeless and independent of the particular culture. The social contract approach is different in that it expects and even encourages variation over time and among cultures. Like faith-based professional ethics, the social contract approach goes outside of medicine for the foundation of its ethical views – but like the existential approach, it is secular.

Thomas Hobbes, John Locke and Jean-Jacques Rousseau developed social contract theory to provide an account of legitimate state authority. They postulated that the state is justified in exercising power to the extent to which its citizens have 'contracted' with it to do so on behalf of their collective welfare. The concept can be extended to address the legitimacy (or lack thereof) of components of the state (like the health professions). In their seminal article, 'Medical professionalism in society', Wynia and his colleagues argue that society 'contracts' with professions – not just the health professions – to protect and promote important societal interests:

Professionalism is a structurally stabilizing, morally protective force in society…societies in different times and places have had in common a need for meritocratic, dedicated subgroups that function to keep private interests and government power in balance through attention to greater social goods. Professions protect not only vulnerable persons but also vulnerable social values…societies may abandon the sick, ignore due process in judging the guilt or innocence of persons accused of a crime…Good civilizations [protect key values] in part by trusting designated groups of people – physicians, lawyers, teachers, journalists, and others – to safeguard the values. (Wynia *et al.* 1999)

Wynia *et al.* define professionalism in terms of three elements: 'devotion' (individual commitment to protecting and advancing health), 'profession' (the promise health professionals make to their patients and to society), and 'negotiation' (give-and-take with government, insurers and health organizations about mutual expectations). While the fundamental commitment to health values, as derived from the existential analysis of illness and care, remain stable, other values will need to be modified over time.

There is no document that establishes the contract between medicine and society, but the concept of a 'social contract' with the health professions is more than a metaphor. According to Creuss and Creuss (2008), the contract may be understood as the sum of laws, regulations, legal precedents and institutional expectations (such as public and private insurance programmes), intangible components like public and patient expectations and commitments made by the health professions:

Under the social contract, the collective expectations of patients, the public, and government of the medical profession constitute a functional definition of medical professionalism and a summary of medicine's professional obligations. (p. 592)

In stable circumstances the underlying 'contract' remains implicit, but when the implicit understandings are violated – as when US health insurers sought to impose a 'gag clause' on physicians to prevent them from telling patients about services that the insurance would not cover – public and professional reaction was swift and strong (Himmelstein and Woolhandler 1995). In the 1980s, changes in social attitudes and gay activism led to the reconceptualization of homosexuality as a normal human variant, not a mental disorder (Bayer 1987). In recent years, patient and family advocates have challenged what they see as stigma and clinical pessimism under the banner of the 'recovery' concept (Anthony 2007). And all industrialized societies are making the demand for health professionals to join in the effort to contain healthcare costs as part of the social contract.

The biopsychosocial model as an ethical vision for mental health professionals

George Engel's biopsychosocial model was not the first effort to conceptualize a holistic approach to patient care, and it will not be the last. But since the publication of his seminal 1977 article in *Science* (Engel 1977) and its 1980 elaboration in the *American Journal of Psychiatry* (Engel 1980), it has been the most widely recognized effort to embrace human complexity and avoid the twin dangers of reductionism and mind–body dualism.

Engel presented the biopsychosocial model as a scientific correction to the biomedical model that prevailed (and still prevails) in medicine. In our view, however, approaching patient care and public health 'biopsychosocially' should also be seen as a statement of the core ethical commitment for the mental health professions. We see the biopsychosocial model as a commitment to respect and appreciate the full range of our beings – synaptic chemistry, personal identity and our participation in family, community, national and even global life – not as a hypothesis or as one theory among many. Engel appears to have recognized the ethical dimensions of the model when he argued that medicine and psychiatry could not meet either their 'scientific tasks or social responsibilities' unless they approached understanding and dealing with human problems in a comprehensive (biopsychosocial) manner. Endorsing a biopsychosocial approach to psychiatry is a way of committing ourselves to recognizing and appreciating human beings in their fullness.

This does not mean that every psychiatrist should give equal attention to each part of the spectrum. Psychiatry needs neuroscientists who focus on synaptic chemistry, psychotherapists who focus on mental process and doctor–patient interaction and social psychiatrists who primarily attend to the impact of social factors. But these specializations must be seen as serving a discipline committed to a holistic understanding of humanity. No one segment has a monopoly on truth.

Similarly, in treating patients it will often be the case that only part of the spectrum needs to be applied. In treating patients with depression, medication alone will fully restore normal function for some, psychotherapy alone will fully restore others, environmental interventions will do the job for still others, and many will require a combination. As a pragmatic, problem-solving profession, we should use the tools best suited to the individual without claiming that the domains to which we are most attached should reign supreme.

The primary intellectual barriers to taking a comprehensive, holistic view of humanity are *reductionism*, 'the philosophic view that complex phenomena are ultimately derived from a single primary principle,' and *mind–body dualism*, 'the doctrine that separates the mental from the somatic' (Engel 1977, p. 130). Dualism sees the body as a machine and issues of emotion and meaning as minimally relevant for understanding and treating disease. Reductionism is a stance of arrogance that claims that one component of knowledge or clinical methodology is an adequate approach to human complexity.

With regard to reductionism, the United States has seen a sharp pendulum swing. After the Second World War, psychoanalytic thinking dominated the leading academic centres. One of us recalls that during his residency training in the 1960s, the revered training director recommended exploratory psychotherapy as the definitive treatment for every patient and referred to medications as 'poisons'! By the 1980s the pendulum was swinging from psychological reductionism towards biological reductionism – from assuming that mental disorders were explained by childhood trauma to assuming that the same disorders were explained by faulty transmitters. The shift to biomedical reductionism was driven in part by advances in neuroscience, but also by the economic interests of pharmaceutical companies and by a trend in public and private insurance to restrict the role of psychiatrists to 'medication management' in an effort to reduce costs.

Reductionism of any form impedes doctor–patient collaboration. Psychological reductionism leads to a search for whom to blame when treatment does not work – either it is the fault of the doctor (deficient empathy) or the patient (deficient motivation). Physical reductionism leads to inadequate attention to the patient's life concerns, as rendered in the joke that 'the operation was a success but unfortunately the patient died'! Failing to appreciate the importance of biological, psychological or social aspects of persons is a failure of compassion and a partial abandonment.

Psychiatry has a unique role within medicine as the specialty most committed to including a full humanistic perspective. Engel intended the biopsychosocial approach to apply to all of medicine, but within medicine psychiatry is the profession most committed to bearing the flag for the values the model embodies. Other medical specialties may make jokes about psychiatry, but they count on mental health clinicians to help them to deal with human complexity.

In our interpretation, the biopsychosocial model is an ethical stance – a commitment to scientific and humanistic openness and against dogmatism. It allows for a pragmatic approach to clinical practice – using those components of current knowledge that are most helpful for an individual patient (Lewis 2007). It allows as well for a pluralistic approach to practice that recognizes that some conditions are best conceptualized primarily in terms of biology, others in terms of psychology or social factors, but it does not succumb to the temptation to retreat into reductionism (Ghaemi 2003). But most importantly, it guides us to a comprehensive appreciation of human complexity, from the molecular to the spiritual, and publicly professes our commitment to this holistic ethic.

Professional ethics, organizational ethics and societal ethics: the Physician Charter

When professional life goes smoothly, we clinicians rarely need to think explicitly about professional ethics. The ethics of professionalism becomes a front burner topic in two circumstances: when members of the profession feel that society is challenging their central commitments or when society fears that the profession is misbehaving.

The Physician Charter (ABIM Foundation *et al.* 2002) was developed by medical leaders from nine countries (Canada, England, France, Holland, Italy, Spain, Sweden, Switzerland and the United States) in response to a shared sense that the health professions were under siege. The distinguished working group apparently felt that the threats to professional values were so clear that the dangers did not have to be specified in any detail beyond this general statement:

Physicians today are experiencing frustration as changes in the healthcare delivery systems in virtually all industrialized countries threaten the very nature and values of medical professionalism … medicine's commitment to the patient is being challenged by external forces of change within our societies. (p. 243)

The Charter presents three fundamental principles followed by a statement of ten professional responsibilities. The first principle, the primacy of patient welfare, is a reaffirmation of medical tradition since Hippocrates. The second principle, support for patient autonomy, is the outcome of a changed social contract negotiated between the health professions and society in the time since the Second World War. The third principle, social justice, is a long-established pillar for public health but will be a new emphasis for some, perhaps many, in mental health. While no rationale is given for adding social justice as a fundamental commitment, it appears to be a response to concern that social forces are skewing health systems in 'unjust' directions, to the belief that physicians must be active in countering unjust trends and to an awareness that society expects the medical profession to help in achieving societal objectives like containing healthcare costs and improving overall access to care.

The ten professional responsibilities are presented as 'commitments': individual and collective professional competence; honesty with patients; patient confidentiality; maintaining appropriate relations with patients; improving quality of care; improving access to care; promoting just distribution of finite resources; advancing scientific knowledge; maintaining trust by managing conflicts of interest; and commitment to collaborating with the profession itself.

The ten commitments are largely familiar and non-controversial. Not surprisingly, a survey of 3500 physicians in the United States showed strong support for the norms proposed in the Charter, ranging from 98% ('Physicians should minimize disparities in care due to patient race or gender' and 'Physicians should be willing to work on quality improvement initiatives'), to 86% ('Physicians should advocate legislation to assure that all people in the United States have health insurance coverage'), to a low of 77% ('Physicians should undergo recertification examinations periodically throughout their career') (Campbell *et al.* 2007). There was more significant variation, however, in terms of self-reported behavioural conformance to the norms. Almost half were aware of an impaired or incompetent colleague but did not take action about the colleague, one third would refer a patient for an unnecessary MRI the patient wanted, and when asked about referring patients to a hypothetical facility they had a financial interest in, a quarter would not inform their patients of the potential conflict of interest.

What is important about the ethics of professionalism?

In training programmes and continuing medical education, the topic of professionalism receives polite attention but, if truth be told, it is often seen as a boring waste of time. We have come to see this reaction – which we have shared in – as a source of insight, not a reason for scolding. There are three main reasons for the reaction.

Statements of professionalism as pious platitudes

We fully agree with the principles and commitments in the Physician Charter, but they are formulated at such an abstract level that they provide only the broadest of frameworks for conducting professional life. Trainees will dutifully agree that mental health professionals should 'maintain appropriate relations with patients' – but they will come to life when one of the group asks, 'One of my patients goes to the same gym I go to – should I stop going? I don't want to do that, but what's the "appropriate" way to handle the situation if I meet him?' Similarly, senior psychiatrists will dutifully agree that 'conflicts of interest should be managed' but will sit on the edge of their chairs and argue vigorously if a colleague asks, 'I believe XYZ is an excellent drug – would it be ethically OK for me to be a speaker for the XYZ company? What would it mean to "manage conflicts of interest" if I join the XYZ speaker bureau?' (Carlat 2007).

The life of ethics is in the details of real situations. Statements of professionalism can only point us in the right direction. As free-standing statements it is easy to see them as pious platitudes. The important work is in bringing the Physician Charter and other manifestos to life by reflecting on how best to apply them in real-life professional circumstances.

Statements of professionalism as powerless ideals

Imagine these scenarios:

A psychiatrist in a community clinic who is scheduled to see patients with serious disorders for 15 minutes every 2 months feels unable to provide good care and feels 'burned out' by the restricted 'med check' role.

A hospital nurse is distressed by the frequency with which patients who are still very symptomatic are discharged to chaotic and unsupportive environments.

A psychotherapist is chronically frustrated by the limited number of sessions the insurance scheme will cover.

If the psychiatrist, nurse and therapist read the Physician Charter assertion that 'market forces, societal pressures, and administrative exigencies must not compromise [the primacy of patient welfare],' they may see the Charter as noble rhetoric with no power to influence the health systems in which they work.

The Charter and other statements of professional ethics are guides for the profession, not contracts with society. Divine law may be enforceable by the Supreme Being, but in complex modern health systems the opportunity to realize professional ideals requires constant negotiation with society. Statements of professionalism are powerless in themselves, but the health professions, if united (Wynia 2008), can influence organizational practices and social policies.

Statements of professionalism as hypocrisy

Society has granted the privileges of self-regulation and profession-driven control to the health professions, but many within wider society and the professions themselves are disappointed with the way these responsibilities have been carried out. Sexual exploitation of patients and financial conflicts of interest that have led to purveying false information about medications have tarnished trust in the mental health professions. Even if the vast majority of professionals have lived up to Justice Cardozo's standard of 'not honesty alone, but the punctilio of an honor the most sensitive' (New York Court of Appeals 1928), widely publicized examples of serious lapses lead some, perhaps many, to see statements of professional ideals as hypocritical fluff.

Conclusions

Given the universal human experience of illness, pain and mortality, it is not surprising that different articulations of health professional ethics – whether derived from religious sources, existential analysis of the care relationship or the contract with society – put a healing orientation and health promotion/disease prevention at the centre. But as healthcare has become more complex and vastly more expensive, hospitals, clinics and other organizations, and those who pay for healthcare, have placed new expectations and demands on health professionals. These are not intended to undermine professional commitment to altruistic healing, but the interaction between professional ideals and new societal demands is laden with strain. For the mental health professions, the major challenge is sustaining the holistic ethical perspective embodied in the biopsychosocial model. The life of contemporary professional ethics lies in negotiation with society about the optimum configuration of professional ideals and other societal values, and how best to apply those ideals in rapidly evolving healthcare systems.

References

ABIM Foundation, ACP-ASIM Foundation, EFIM (2002). Medical professionalism in the new millennium: a physician charter. *Annals of Internal Medicine* **136**(3), 243–246.

Anthony W A (2007). *Toward a Vision of Recovery*. Boston: Boston University Center for Psychiatric Rehabilitation.

Bayer R (1987). *Homosexuality and American Society: The Politics of Diagnosis*. Princeton: Princeton University Press.

Campbell E G, Regan S, Gruen R L (2007). Professionalism in medicine: results of a national survey of physicians. *Annals of Internal Medicine* **147**, 795–802.

Carlat D (25 November 2007). Dr. Drug Rep. *New York Times*. www.nytimes.com/2007/11/25/magazine/25memoir-t.html?pagewanted=1. Last accessed 20 April 2010.

Creuss R L, Creuss S R (2008). Expectations and obligations: professionalism and medicine's social contract with society. *Perspectives in Biology and Medicine* **51**, 579–598.

Engel G L (1977). The need for a new medical model: a challenge for biomedicine. *Science* **196**, 129–136.

Engel G L (1980). The clinical application of the biopsychosocial model. *American Journal of Psychiatry* **137**, 535–544.

Ghaemi S N (2003). *The Concepts of Psychiatry: A Pluralistic Approach to the Mind and Mental Illness*. Baltimore: Johns Hopkins Press.

Heritage Illustrated Dictionary of the English Language (1979). Boston: Houghton Mifflin Press.

Himmelstein D, Woolhandler S (1995). Extreme risk – the new corporate proposition for physicians. *New England Journal of Medicine* **333**, 1706–1708.

Keown D W (2004). Buddhism and bioethics. In J F Peppin, M J Cherry (eds.) *Religious Perspectives in Bioethics*. London and New York: Taylor & Francis Press, pp. 173–188.

Lewis B (2007). The biopsychosocial model and philosophic pragmatism: is George Engel a pragmatist? *Philosophy, Psychiatry, & Psychology* **14**, 299–310.

New York Court of Appeals (1928). *Morton H. Meinhard v Walter J. Salmon*. http://en.wikisource.org/wiki/Meinhard_v._Salmon. Last accessed 20 April 2010.

Pellegrino E M (2006). Toward a reconstruction of medical morality. *American Journal of Bioethics* **6**, 65–71.

Pellegrino E D, Thomasma D C (1993). *The Virtues in Medical Practice*. New York: Oxford University Press.

Sulmasy D P (1999). What is an oath and why should physicians swear one? *Theoretical Medicine and Bioethics* **20**, 329–346.

Sulmasy D P (2009). Spirituality, religion, and clinical care. *Chest* **135**, 1634–1642.

Veatch R M (2001). The impossibility of a morality internal to medicine. *Journal of Medicine and Philosophy* **26**, 621–642.

Wynia M K (2008). The short history and tenuous future of medical professionalism. *Perspectives in Biology and Medicine* **51**, 565–578.

Wynia M K, Latham S R, Kao A C, Berg J W, Emanuel L L (1999). Medical professionalism in society. *New England Journal of Medicine* **341**, 1611–1616.

Training in professionalism

Vikram Jha, Zeryab Setna and Trudie Roberts

Editors' introduction

Professionalism can be learnt using observational or narrative models. In addition, being mentored, role modelling and being an apprentice can all be used to learn about professional skills as well as values, attitudes and beliefs. The components of professionalism may be clear, depending upon whatever definitions are used, and it is easier to learn and teach some components when compared with others. Jha *et al.* emphasize the need for formal training in professionalism and argue that the evaluation of professionalism has not received the same attention in the curriculum as has the evaluation of knowledge and skills. The informal process of socialization from medical school through psychiatric training has been described as a hidden curriculum, and these authors argue that this is not the best way to learn about professionalism. Furthermore, professionalism should be seen as a developmental process rather than as a static one. The role of assessment in learning to become a professional needs to be emphasized. Jha *et al.* point out that in order to understand professional behaviours, the underlying cognitive determinants of such behaviour must be understood. The related question is whether these cognitive determinants are changeable and, if so, what factors can bring this (change) about. Jha *et al.* use the theory of planned behaviour, which argues that an individual's behaviour is underpinned by their cognitions as the behaviour is primarily dependent on the intention to perform the particular behaviour, which is in turn influenced by a number of factors. Such an approach can provide outcomes which may be measurable and consistent. Moreover, this approach may also provide a focus on components of professionalism rather than a totally abstract concept. Such an approach can easily be divided into constituent components, and consequently training and learning can become much more focused.

Introduction

There is universal acknowledgement of the importance of training in professionalism in medical education (General Medical Council 2001, ABIM Foundation *et al.* 2002, General Medical Council 2002, Cruess *et al.* 2009). Formal evaluation of professionalism has emerged relatively recently as a major agenda for undergraduate, postgraduate and continuing medical education compared with evaluation of knowledge and skills (Papadakis *et al.* 1999). There is now a substantial body of literature on the determinants of professionalism and on methods to develop and assess professional attributes and behaviours in medicine (Jha *et al.*

Professionalism in Mental Healthcare: Experts, Expertise and Expectations, ed. Dinesh Bhugra and Amit Malik. Published by Cambridge University Press. © Cambridge University Press 2011.

2007a, Parker *et al.* 2008, Wilkinson *et al.* 2009). However, interventions designed to promote professionalism still have major limitations, and the evidence for their effectiveness is limited (Jha *et al.* 2007a).

Definitions of professionalism are abundant in the literature; these represent expert opinion (ABIM Foundation *et al.* 2002, Hilton and Slotnick 2005, Royal College of Physicians 2005) or research-led conceptualization of professionalism (Jha *et al.* 2005, Wagner *et al.* 2007). Most of the measures and interventions designed to facilitate professionalism evaluate behaviours related to professionalism rather than attitudes (Jha *et al.* 2007a). These proxy measures of attitudes describe choices that an individual makes, manifested as the behaviour witnessed, but they do not always reflect on how he or she arrived at the decision (Ginsburg *et al.* 2000). A measure of attitudes and beliefs that underpin professional behaviour may provide more insight into these complex cognitions rather than simple observation of behaviours. For the purpose of this chapter, therefore, we define professionalism as a construct of attitudes and beliefs that will determine whether an individual will engage in professional or unprofessional behaviour. This approach to professionalism is now being advocated by researchers in the field (Jha *et al.* 2007b, Archer *et al.* 2008) as a means to facilitate understanding and training in professionalism.

Four main issues are discussed in this chapter: the need for formal training in professionalism; the evidence for effectiveness of training in professionalism; the role of assessment in driving learning to become a professional; and the theoretical underpinning of interventions designed to facilitate professionalism in medicine.

The need for formal training in professionalism

Professionalism-related issues form the basis for the majority of complaints against doctors (General Medical Council 2002, Papadakis *et al.* 2004). Regulating bodies such as the General Medical Council (GMC) and the American Board of Internal Medicine (ABIM) now explicitly state that training to become a professional must include not just acquisition of professional knowledge and skills, but also of appropriate attitudes and behaviours (GMC 2001, ABIM Foundation *et al.* 2002, GMC 2002). There is evidence that those who demonstrate poor professional attributes as students are more likely to do so when they are in practice. For example, Sierles *et al.* (1980) reported that students who cheat during medical school are significantly more likely to cheat in practice. Papadakis *et al.* (2004) found that problematic behaviour in medical school was associated with increased risk of subsequent disciplinary action by a state board. In addition, there are reports that suggest that high levels of moral reasoning amongst residents (Rowley *et al.* 2000) and students (Meetz *et al.* 1988) are associated with higher levels of clinical performance.

However, evaluation of professionalism has not received the same attention in the curriculum as evaluation of knowledge and skills (Papadakis *et al.* 1999). There is therefore a limited body of literature in the area of teaching and assessment of professionalism compared with the literature on teaching and assessment of knowledge and skills. Often, it is assumed that learning about and development of attitudes, behaviours and values related to professionalism can take place through the 'hidden curriculum' (Jackson 1966). This involves an informal process of socialization commencing at medical school and extending through to postgraduate training and subsequent practice of medicine, rather than in more formal settings such as lectures or tutorials (Stern 1998, Swick *et al.* 1999). The hidden curriculum should now be regarded as inadequate in promoting professionalism (Gaiser 2009) as it relies on students learning about professionalism through informal means, such as observing role models and learning from experiences on the wards or clinics and even in their social life. Learning about professionalism using role models does not guarantee excellence (Ber and Alroy 2002). Moreover, the faculty serving as role models are often unaware of their exact role in promoting professionalism (Gaiser 2009). There may be poor role models (Lingard *et al.* 1998), and how students distinguish them from good role models is poorly researched. Consequently, a number of medical schools now perceive the need for more explicit teaching of medical professionalism within their curriculum (Goldstein *et al.* 2006, Goldie 2008). Such programmes need to be introduced relatively early in the curriculum in order to identify problems sooner (Loeser and Papadakis 2000); thus, students with problems related to professionalism may then have time to undergo remediation, mentoring and targeted teaching in order to improve some aspects of professional behaviour, such as communication and maturity (Loeser and Papadakis 2000). In addition, there is increasing emphasis on the incorporation of formal training in professionalism for postgraduates (Gaiser 2009), with residencies in the United States (Gaiser 2009) and Royal Colleges in the UK (RCP 2005) supporting the promotion of professionalism amongst its trainees and practising clinicians.

It is believed that professionalism is a developmental process rather than a fixed, unchanging concept (Baldwin and Bunch 2000). More recent definitions of professionalism have included the concept of 'protoprofessionalism' to describe the 'lengthy state in which the learner develops the skills and knowledge, and gains the experience needed to acquire professionalism' (Hilton and Slotnick 2005, p. 59). Protoprofessionalism may therefore be considered to be the phase that leads to professionalism after a prolonged period of learning, instruction and self-reflection (Hilton and Slotnick 2005). In addition, attitudes – particularly towards ethical and moral issues – may change or decline as students progress through the medical curriculum (Woloschuk *et al.* 2004). The belief that students will be admitted to medical school equipped with a complete set of values and professional skills is no longer tenable. In addition, if the development of professionalism is as prolonged as some researchers suggest (Hilton and Slotnick 2005), then the rationale for training in professionalism to extend into postgraduate and indeed continuing education becomes even more relevant.

The evidence for effectiveness of training in professionalism

There is evidence in the medical education literature of how medical schools are currently integrating the teaching of professionalism into their formal curricula (Goldstein *et al.* 2006, Goldie 2008, Parker *et al.* 2008). The methods of teaching reported in such curricula include introductory lectures on professionalism at the start of medical school followed by sequential discussions and teaching about professional behaviour throughout the curriculum (Gibson *et al.* 2000, Fincher 2001). Formal personal and professional development (PPD) programmes which are incorporated within the curriculum to foster the development of professional competencies and attributes in students are also reported (Gordon 2003, Parker *et al.* 2008). These include teaching on communication skills, humane care, self-care, ethics and health law and medical humanities (Gordon 2003). Individual stand-alone courses that specifically target teaching of professional behaviour have also been described as a means of teaching professionalism. These courses either address professionalism as a comprehensive concept (Hafferty 2002) or concentrate on specific areas of professionalism, such as ethics teaching for undergraduates (Browne *et al.* 1995), patient-centred medicine for residents (Yeheskel *et al.* 2000) or communication with patients (Ang 2002).

Most of the teaching of professionalism reported in the literature addresses knowledge, skills and behaviours associated with professionalism (Jha *et al.* 2007a). For example, there are reports of teaching about appropriate and inappropriate professional behaviour (Gibson *et al.* 2000, Ber and Alroy 2002), teaching about knowledge of professional attributes such as humane qualities (Howe 2002), patient-centredness (Yeheskel *et al.* 2000), compassion and humility (Wear 1998) and ethical practice (Browne *et al.* 1995). Teaching of skills related to professionalism, such as communication skills (Ang 2002), is also reported in the literature. There are few programmes that teach or evaluate attitudes towards professionalism; the programmes that have been reported address specific components of professionalism such as ethical issues (Goldie *et al.* 2002) or socio-cultural issues (Tang *et al.* 2002) rather than attitudes towards professionalism as a whole. There appears to be no attempt by these teaching programmes to operationalize or clearly define the concepts of professionalism, thereby leaving a gap in medical school curricula in the area of facilitating the development of attitudes towards professionalism.

Jha *et al.* (2007a) found no interventions that reported changes in attitudes towards professionalism in the long term. There were only two interventions that measured attitude change longitudinally. Of these, Goldie *et al.* (2002) measured the impact of ethics teaching on attitudes towards ethical dilemmas in a cohort of students over 3 years. They reported an improvement in attitude scores after 1 year, but no change after that. Goldie *et al.* (2003) measured attitudes and potential behaviour with regard to whistle-blowing in students pre- and post-Year 1, post-Year 3 and post-Year 5, but they failed to report any significant change in attitudes. There is therefore little evidence of interventions that are effective in changing attitudes to professionalism in the long term. Moreover, few studies (Moore *et al.* 1994, Boenink *et al.* 2005) reported interventions addressing professionalism as a whole, and no studies referred to the behaviour change literature when describing the theoretical framework of interventions aimed at impacting on student attitudes. These weaknesses limit the evidence for practical and effective interventions to facilitate professional attitudes.

The role of assessment in driving learning to become a professional

In addition to formalizing the teaching of professionalism, there is also recognition of the need to formalize the assessment of professionalism. This may represent one way of informing medical students and even society that acquisition of appropriate attitudes to professionalism during medical education is important (Boon and Turner 2004). There is evidence that assessment drives learning, and lack of formal assessment may undermine the impact of teaching by making students think that it is not as important as other areas that are more rigorously assessed, such as knowledge and clinical skills (Goldie *et al.* 2002). Formal assessment also encourages growth of students in the direction of professionalism (Bickel 1991) and allows educators to monitor the acquisition of these attitudes and behaviours amongst learners. Equally, formal assessment helps to evaluate the quality and effectiveness of programmes designed to promote the development of professionalism (Arnold 2002).

The assessment strategies described in the literature (Veloski *et al.* 2005, Jha *et al.* 2007a) evaluate the knowledge of and attitudes to professionalism, as well as the application of this knowledge/these attitudes in practice. This application is assessed through observation of skills and behaviours in classroom and real-world settings. Assessment in the workplace reflects the notion that learning and assessment go hand in hand (Billet 2002). It also incorporates the principles of the situated learning theory (Lave and Wenger 1991, Steinert 2009), which suggests that learning occurs best in the context to which it is applied. A range of workplace-based assessment measures are being used, particularly in postgraduate specialist training, to evaluate the development of professional skills amongst trainees (CIPHER 2007, Norcini and Burch 2007). A number of these measures evaluate professional behaviours, for example the mini-CEX and multisource feedback (Wilkinson *et al.* 2009). The effectiveness of these tools in capturing the aspects of professionalism being assessed is becoming established (Wilkinson *et al.* 2009); moreover, the evaluation of how these tools facilitate learning is being researched (Setna *et al.*, unpublished data).

The theoretical underpinning of interventions designed to facilitate professionalism in medicine: the theory of planned behaviour

There is an emerging consensus on the component parts of professionalism (Wilkinson *et al.* 2009); however, these components are still described using such terms as altruism, integrity and honesty, which are difficult to operationalize or evaluate (Jha *et al.* 2005, RCP 2005, Wagner *et al.* 2007, Holtman 2008). There is also an expanding body of literature on interventions and methods designed to teach and/or assess medical professionalism (Arnold 2002, Lynch *et al.* 2004, Veloski *et al.* 2005, Jha *et al.* 2007a). However, most of these interventions have been developed without using an appropriate theoretical framework (Rees and Knight 2007) and have relied on measures of specific behaviours related to professionalism, with little regard to the determinants of the behaviours (Jha *et al.* 2007a, Rees and Knight 2007). These interventions also do not focus specifically on measures of attitudes, strategies to change attitudes or associations between attitudes and future practising behaviour.

A systematic review of measures of professionalism (Jha *et al.* 2007a) highlighted the need for an appropriate paradigm for the teaching and assessment of professionalism in medicine. To understand professional behaviour, it is necessary to explore the cognitive determinants of that behaviour (Jha *et al.* 2005, Wagner *et al.* 2007). Theory-based interventions are hypothesized as being more effective in changing behaviour than atheoretical ones (Grimshaw *et al.* 2002, Eccles *et al.* 2005, Eccles *et al.* 2007). Indeed, conceptual models represent a set of concepts (words describing mental images of phenomena) and the propositions (statements about the concepts) that integrate the former into a meaningful configuration (Fawcett 1989). Conceptual models are rarely static, and many evolve as evidence emerges. Then, a more established view of the world becomes a theory, which has a narrower focus and can be experimentally refuted (Popper 2002). More importantly, conceptual models and theories lay the grounds for hypotheses that can be tested in rigorous research.

The Theory of Planned Behaviour (TPB) (Ajzen 1985) provides a framework to understand the association between a behaviour and the cognitive attributes that underpin it. It is among the most used theories for studying behaviours in individuals (Glanz *et al.* 1997). In the past decade, it has been one of the most used theories for studying healthcare providers' behaviours (Conner and Sparks 2005, Godin *et al.* 2008). Health behaviours that have been targeted by TPB applications include drug use (McMillan and Conner 2003), sexual behaviour (Albarracin *et al.* 2001) and dietary behaviours (Conner *et al.* 2001). The TPB has been able to explain considerable variation in behavioural intentions across these behaviours (Conner and Sparks 2005). The TPB (Figure 14.1) is a deliberative

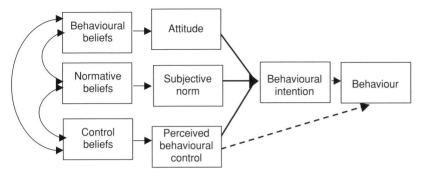

Figure 14.1 Theory of Planned Behaviour (TPB) (Ajzen 1985)

processing model that explains how an individual's behaviour is underpinned by his or her cognitions. In brief, the model states that behaviour is primarily dependent on the intention to perform the particular behaviour; intention is determined by three variables: attitude towards the behaviour, subjective norm and perceived behavioural control. Attitude towards the behaviour is a function of behavioural beliefs (performing the behaviour leads to some consequence) and beliefs on outcomes of the behaviour (evaluations of consequence); subjective norm is a function of normative beliefs (perceptions of specific significant others' preferences about whether one should or should not engage in a particular behaviour) and motivation to comply (extent to which one wishes to comply with significant others' expectations); perceived behavioural control is influenced by beliefs concerning whether one has access to the resources or opportunities to perform the behaviour successfully and perception of factors with power to facilitate or inhibit the performance of the behaviour. According to the TPB, the more favourable the attitude and subjective norm and the greater the perceived behavioural control, the stronger the individual's intention to perform the behaviour under consideration (Ajzen 1985).

There are suggestions of the possible application of the TPB as a framework within which training and assessment of professionalism may be developed (Jha *et al.* 2007b, Rees and Knight 2007, Archer *et al.* 2008). These suggestions are based on the following arguments:

1. The application of the TPB framework provides some understanding of the possible determinants of professional and unprofessional behaviour in medicine. One of the major criticisms of research on professionalism is the inability of measures to address professionalism as a comprehensive concept rather than individual behaviours (Lynch *et al.* 2004, Veloski *et al.* 2005, Jha *et al.* 2007a). The TPB allows the development of measures that incorporate different facets of professional and unprofessional behaviour in medicine.

2. The TPB variables offer theory-based outcomes that could provide consistency between different institutions designing courses on professionalism (Archer *et al.* 2008). For example, attitudes could be targeted through self-assessment (Jha *et al.* 2007b) and formal and informal discussions around the consequences of professional and unprofessional behaviour. These are particularly relevant with regards to training in patient safety, the consequences of medical error and the reduction of patient complaints and litigation. The influence of positive and negative role models and the impact of societal norms on professionalism-related behaviours have been recognized (Pololi *et al.* 2001, Stephenson *et al.* 2006). Jha *et al.* (2007b) also found normative

beliefs to be a strong predictor of intention to behave professionally. The ease or difficulties associated with behaving professionally are linked with the culture within which students and doctors work, as well as the provision of reinforcement and feedback on their behaviour (Bandura *et al.* 1977). Targeting behavioural control through encouragement of expression of individual attitudes, adequate role modelling of professionalism and structured feedback on professional behaviour may enhance professionalism amongst students and trainees and also increase their satisfaction with their performance (Multon *et al.* 1991, Archer *et al.* 2008).

3. Having a standardized measure is important because it will facilitate the comparison between similar studies, make it possible to carry out a systematic review in this area, help to inform policy-makers in the implementation of professionalism behaviours in medical students and, most importantly, contribute to the elaboration of a theoretical base for translating professionalism into medical practice.

Future directions

Teaching about professionalism should be directed not only at influencing professional behaviour, but should also address attitudes and beliefs related to these behaviours. The popularity of the TPB framework in designing behavioural interventions is related to the idea that changing a person's beliefs will lead to changes in the other components of the theory, such as attitudes and behaviour (Conner and Sparks 2005). Jha *et al.* (2007b) have developed a measure using the TPB framework to explore medical students' intention to behave professionally or unprofessionally. They have reported strong correlation between behavioural intention and beliefs that may underpin professionalism-related behaviour; these beliefs may also have an influence in predicting intentions to engage in these behaviours.

Any teaching programme on professionalism should include tapping into influences of likely outcomes of behaving professionally or unprofessionally, as well as the influence of significant referent groups such as peers and role models on professional behaviour. Influences related to past behaviour and the possible impact of past experiences related to the particular aspect of professionalism being taught may also be important in influencing behavioural change.

References

ABIM Foundation, ACP-ASIM Foundation, EFIM (2002). Medical professionalism in the new millennium: a physician charter. *Annals of Internal Medicine* **136**(3), 243–246.

Ajzen I (1985). From intentions to action: a theory of planned behaviour. In J Kuhl, J Beckmann (eds.) *Action-Control: From Cognition to Behaviour*. Heidelberg: Springer, pp. 11–39.

Albarracin D, Johnson B T, Fishbein M, Muellerleile P A (2001). Theories of reasoned action and planned behaviour as models of condom use: a meta-analysis. *Psychological Bulletin* **127**, 142–161.

Ang M (2002). Advanced communication skills: conflict management and persuasion. *Academic Medicine* **77**, 1166.

Archer R, Elder W, Hustedde C, Milam A, Joyce J (2008). The theory of planned behaviour in medical education: a model for integrating professionalism training. *Medical Education* **42**, 771–777.

Arnold L (2002). Assessing professional behaviour: yesterday, today and tomorrow. *Academic Medicine* **77**, 502–515.

Baldwin D C, Jr, Bunch W H (2000). Moral reasoning, professionalism, and the teaching of ethics to orthopaedic surgeons. *Clinical Orthopaedics and Related Research* **378**, 97–103.

Bandura A, Adams N E, Beyer J (1977). Cognitive processes mediating behavioural change. *Journal of Personality and Social Psychology* **35**, 125–139.

Ber R, Alroy G (2002). Teaching professionalism with the aid of trigger films. *Medical Teacher* **24**, 528–531.

Bickel J (1991). Medical students' professional ethics: defining the problems and developing resources. *Academic Medicine* **66**, 726–729.

Billet S (2002). Guided learning at work. In D Boud, J Garrick (eds.) *Understanding Learning at Work*. New York: Routledge, pp. 151–164.

Boenink A D, de Jonge P, Smal K, Oderwald A, van Tilburg W (2005). The effects of teaching medical professionalism by means of vignettes: an exploratory study. *Medical Teacher* **27**(5), 429–432.

Boon K, Turner J (2004). Ethical and professional conduct of medical students: review of current assessment measures and controversies. *Journal of Medical Ethics* **30**, 221–226.

Browne A, Carpenter C, Cooledge C, *et al.* (1995). Bridging the professions: an integrated and interdisciplinary approach to teaching health care ethics. *Academic Medicine* **70**(11), 1002–1005.

Centre for Innovation in Professional Health Education and Research (CIPHER) (2007). *Review of Work-Based Assessment Methods*. Sydney: University of Sydney.

Conner M, Kirk S F L, Cade J E, Barrett J H (2001). Why do women use dietary supplements? The use of the theory of planned behaviour to explore beliefs about their use. *Social Science and Medicine* **52**, 621–633.

Conner M, Sparks P (2005). Theory of planned behaviour and health behaviour. In M Conner, P Norman (eds.) *Predicting Health Behaviour*. Milton Keynes: Open University Press, pp. 170–222.

Cruess R L, Cruess S R, Steinert Y (2009). *Teaching Medical Professionalism*. New York: Cambridge University Press.

Eccles M, Grimshaw J, Walker A, Johnston M, Pitts N (2005). Changing the behavior of healthcare professionals: the use of theory in promoting the uptake of research findings. *Journal of Clinical Epidemiology* **58**, 107–112.

Eccles M P, Grimshaw J M, Johnston M, *et al.* (2007). Applying psychological theories to evidence-based clinical practice: identifying factors predictive of managing upper respiratory tract infections without antibiotics. *Implementation Science* **2**, 26.

Fawcett J (1989). *Conceptual Models and Theories: Analysis and Evaluation of Conceptual Models of Nursing*. Philadelphia, PA: F.A. Davis Company.

Fincher R E (2001). A longitudinal approach to teaching and assessing professional attitudes and behaviours in medical school. *Academic Medicine* **76**, 505–506.

Gaiser R R (2009). The teaching of professionalism during residency: why it is failing and a suggestion to improve its success. *Anesthesia & Analgesia* **108**, 948–954.

General Medical Council (2001). *Good Medical Practice*. London: GMC.

General Medical Council (2002). *Tomorrow's Doctors: Recommendations on Undergraduate Medical Education*. London: GMC.

Gibson D D, Coldwell L L, Kiewitt S F (2000). Creating a culture of professionalism: an integrated approach. *Academic Medicine* **75**, 509.

Ginsburg S, Regehr G, Hatala R, *et al.* (2000). Context, conflict and resolution: a new conceptual framework for evaluating professionalism. *Academic Medicine* **75**(10 Suppl), S6–S11.

Glanz K, Lewis F, Rimer B (1997). Theory, research and practice in health behavior and health education. In K Glanz, F Lewis, B Rimer (eds.) *Health Behavior and Health Education: Theory, Research and Practice*. San Francisco: Jossey-Bass, pp. 22–40.

Godin G, Belanger-Gravel A, Eccles M, Grimshaw J (2008). Healthcare professionals' intentions and behaviours: a systematic review of studies based on social cognitive theories. *Implementation Science* **3**, 36.

Goldie J (2008). Integrating professionalism teaching into undergraduate medical education in the UK setting. *Medical Teacher* **30**, 513–527.

Goldie J, Schwartz L, McConnachie A, Morrison J (2002). The impact of three years' ethics teaching in an integrated medical curriculum, on students' proposed behaviour on meeting ethical dilemmas. *Medical Education* **36**, 489–497.

Goldie J, Schwartz L, McConnachie A, Morrison J (2003). Students' attitudes and potential behaviour with regard to whistle blowing as they pass through a modern medical curriculum. *Medical Education* **37**, 368–375.

Goldstein E A, Maestas R R, Fryer-Edwards K, *et al.* (2006). Professionalism in medical education: an institutional challenge. *Academic Medicine* **81**, 871–876.

Gordon G (2003). Fostering students' personal and professional development in medicine: a new framework for PPD. *Medical Education* **37**, 341–349.

Grimshaw J M, Eccles M P, Walker A E, Thomas R E (2002). Changing physicians' behavior: what works and thoughts on getting more things to work. *Journal of Continuing Education in the Health Professions* **22**, 237–243.

Hafferty F W (2002). What medical students know about professionalism. *The Mount Sinai Journal of Medicine* **69**, 385–397.

Hilton S R, Slotnick H B (2005). Protoprofessionalism: how professionalisation occurs across the continuum of medical education. *Medical Education* **39**, 58–65.

Holtman M C (2008). A theoretical sketch of medical professionalism as a normative complex. *Advances in Health Science Education* **13**, 233–245.

Howe A (2002). Professional development in undergraduate medical education. *Medical Education* **34**, 353–359.

Jackson P (1966). The students' world. *The Elementary School Journal* **66**, 353.

Jha V, Bekker H L, Duffy S R G, Roberts T E (2005). Perceptions of professionalism in medicine: a qualitative study. *Medical Education* **40**, 1027–1036.

Jha V, Bekker H L, Duffy S R G, Roberts T E (2007a). A systematic review of studies assessing and facilitating attitudes towards professionalism in medicine. *Medical Education* **41**, 822–829.

Jha V, Bekker H L, Pell G, Conner M, Roberts T E (2007b). Influence of attitudes and beliefs on prediction of medical students' intentions to behave professionally. *Abstracts of Association of Medical Education in Europe (AMEE) Conference*, Trondheim, 134.

Lave J, Wenger E (1991). *Situated Learning. Legitimate Peripheral Participation*. Cambridge: Cambridge University Press.

Lingard L, Reznick R, Espin S, Regehr G, DeVito I (2002). Team communications in the operating room: talk patterns, sites of tension, and implications for novices. *Academic Medicine* 77, 232–237.

Loeser H, Papadakis M (2000). Promoting and assessing professionalism in the first two years of medical school. *Academic Medicine* 75, 509–510.

Lynch D C, Surdyk P M, Eiser A R (2004). Assessing professionalism: a review of the literature. *Medical Teacher* 26, 366–373.

McMillan B, Conner M (2003). Applying an extended version of the theory of planned behaviour to illicit drug use among students. *Journal of Applied Social Psychology* 33, 1662–1683.

Meetz H K, Bebeau M J, Thoma S J (1988). The validity and reliability of a clinical performance rating scale. *Journal of Dental Education* 52(6), 290–297.

Moore G T, Block S D, Style C B, Mitchell R (1994). The influence of the New Pathway Curriculum on Harvard medical students. *Academic Medicine* 69, 983–989.

Multon K D, Brown S D, Lent R W (1991). Relation of self-efficacy beliefs to academic outcomes: a meta-analytic investigation. *Journal of Counselling Psychology* 38, 30–38.

Norcini J J, Burch V (2007). Workplace-based assessment as an educational tool: AMEE Guide No. 31. *Medical Teacher* 29(9), 855–871.

Papadakis M A, Osborn E H, Cooke M, Healy K (1999). A strategy for the detection and evaluation of unprofessional behaviour in medical students. *Academic Medicine* 74, 980–990.

Papadakis M A, Hodgson C S, Teherani A, Kohatsu N D (2004). Unprofessional behaviour in medical school is associated with subsequent disciplinary action by a State Medical Board. *Academic Medicine* 79(3), 244–249.

Parker M, Luke H, Zhang J, Wilkinson D, Peterson R, Ozolins L (2008). The 'pyramid of professionalism': seven years of experience with an integrated program of teaching, developing and assessing professionalism among medical students. *Academic Medicine* 83, 733–741.

Pololi L, Frankel R M, Clay M, Jobe A C (2001). One year's experience with a programme to facilitate personal and professional development in medical students using reflection groups. *Education for Health* 14, 36–49.

Popper K (2002). *The Logic of Scientific Discovery*. London: Routledge Classics.

Rees C E, Knight L V (2007). The trouble with assessing students' professional behaviors: theoretical insights from socio-cognitive psychology. *Academic Medicine* 82, 46–50.

Rowley B D, Baldwin D C, Jr, Bay RC, Cannula M (2000). Can professional values be taught? A look at residency training. *Clinical Orthopaedics* 378, 110–114.

Royal College of Physicians (2005). *Doctors in Society: Medical Professionalism in a Changing World*. Report of a working party of the Royal College of Physicians of London. London: RCP.

Sierles F, Hendrickx I, Circle S (1980). Cheating in medical school. *Journal of Medical Education* 55(2), 124–125.

Steinert Y (2009). Educational theory and strategies for teaching and learning professionalism. In R L Cruess, S R Cruess, Y Steinert (eds.) *Teaching Medical Professionalism*. New York: Cambridge University Press, pp. 31–52.

Stephenson A E, Adshead L E, Higgs R H (2006). The teaching of professional attitudes within UK medical schools: reported difficulties and good practice. *Medical Education* 40, 1072–1080.

Stern D T (1998). In search of the informal curriculum: when and where professional values are taught. *Academic Medicine* 73, S28–S30.

Swick H M, Szenas P, Danoff D, Whitcomb M E (1999). Teaching professionalism in undergraduate medical education. *Journal of the American Medical Association* 282, 830–832.

Tang T S, Fantone J C, Bozynski M E A, Adams B S (2002). Implementation and evaluation of an undergraduate sociocultural medicine program. *Academic Medicine* 77, 578–585.

Veloski J J, Fields S K, Boex J R, Blank L L (2005). Measuring professionalism: a review of studies with instruments reported in the literature between 1982 and 2002. *Academic Medicine* **80**, 366–370.

Wagner P, Hendrich J, Moseley G, Hudson V (2007). Defining medical professionalism: a qualitative study. *Medical Education* **41**, 288–294.

Wear D (1998). On white coats and professional development: the formal and hidden curricula. *Annals of Internal Medicine* **129**, 734–737.

Wilkinson T J, Wade W B, Knock L D (2009). A blueprint to assess professionalism: results of a systematic review. *Academic Medicine* **84**, 551–558.

Woloschuk W, Harasym P H, Temple W (2004). Attitude change during medical school: a cohort study. *Medical Education* **38**, 522–534.

Yeheskel A, Biderman A, Borkan J M, Herman J (2000). A course for teaching patient-centered medicine to family medicine residents. *Academic Medicine* **75**, 494–497.

Chapter 15

Expertise and medical professionalism

Kathy M. Vincent and Allan Tasman

Editors' introduction

Experts are individuals who have attained that status after a long period of training and experience. It is important that suitable training is available so that individuals can develop their skills, gain confidence and develop their beliefs and attitudes in the right direction. It is essential that, having obtained levels of expertise, the clinician not only keeps up-to-date and maintains standards of good clinical practice, but also continues to practise in a professionally prescribed manner. Vincent and Tasman point out that with rapidly changing medical knowledge, it is crucial that medical professionalism should include maintaining up-to-date knowledge as an important component. Equally important is the role of the professional organizations and societies in ensuring that the public is protected by high standards of medical expertise which is kept at par with changes. Vincent and Tasman argue that expertise and professionalism are inextricably linked. Medical professionalism is demonstrated by what the physicians do with patients and their communities. Medical professionalism consists of all the behaviours necessary to be worthy of public trust. The feeling of disenfranchisement felt by doctors in the United States and elsewhere is linked to the removal of some of the traditional privileges which have been granted by society. Needless to say that these and other such privileges cannot and should not be taken for granted. To retain public trust doctors must maintain standards. A competency-based framework is a step forward. By agreeing to the identification of common terms and definitions, competency expectations can be shared across the continuum of medical education. Competencies in licensing and credentialing can provide a way forward in maintaining high standards of care and healthcare delivery.

Introduction

The relationship between the medical profession and society is changing owing to a number of forces in and outside medicine. Medical knowledge and practice skills are rapidly increasing with new scientific discoveries in genetics, bioengineering, informatics and technology. Medical professionalism should include maintaining an up-to-date knowledge and skills base and is core to maintaining the trust bestowed upon physicians by society, which is central to the doctor–patient relationship. Professional institutions – including medical schools, teaching hospitals, professional societies and organizations and licensing bodies – have a role in protecting the public by setting and maintaining standards for physicians. Doctors have a responsibility to maintain their medical expertise and to demonstrate professionalism as

Professionalism in Mental Healthcare: Experts, Expertise and Expectations, ed. Dinesh Bhugra and Amit Malik. Published by Cambridge University Press. © Cambridge University Press 2011.

part of their contract with society. Expertise and professionalism are therefore inextricably linked. This chapter will review how this issue has been reflected in the various components of medical training, accreditation and practice in the United States.

Definition of medical professionalism

Defining professionalism is not an easy task. Some would say that professionalism is more easily described than defined. There are, however, distinct attributes that are identified as professional, and these personal characteristics and behaviours must be taught to the next generation of physicians and assessed in those currently in practice. A brief review of this issue will set the stage for the discussion of the intersection of professionalism and expertise. Although this has been covered elsewhere in this book, it is important to contextualize it here.

To define professionalism, one must understand the common features of a profession.

Using a sociological framework, a profession is conceptualized by the work done by its members. A profession requires formalized education, produces scholarly writings for dialogue about its ideals and enjoys respect by the public (Lathan 2002). A profession has a specialized body of knowledge, possesses recognized expertise and functions with a certain autonomy and self-regulation granted by society as long as the profession meets its responsibilities to the general population (Cohen 2006). For example, medical professionals in most countries establish and monitor their educational training standards, maintain licensure processes and have disciplinary mechanisms, and in return they are expected to assure that physicians are qualified to practise the specialty.

Current views of a profession have also considered the moral and ethical value of the work performed. Some view a professional as an advocate for social values, making a profession a way of life or a calling, not just an occupation (Swick 2000). Talcott Parsons, a well-known twentieth-century sociologist, believed the existence of a profession in moral terms was tied to the work done by its members. According to the Parsonian view, physicians use their expert authority to negotiate and mediate between patients and society (Lathan 2002). For example, doctors can tell patients not to drink and drive. They gain authority on the basis of their medical expertise. Professional standards are necessary because of physician authority and patient vulnerability in this relationship.

Medical professionalism is demonstrated by what the physicians do with patients and their communities. This is how the physician fulfils the contract with society. The values that have been associated with the profession of medicine include service, altruism, duty, advocacy, respect, honesty, integrity, excellence and accountability, among others (Stern 2006, MacKenzie 2007).

Another way to define medical professionalism is to say that it consists of all the behaviours necessary to be worthy of public trust. These include responding to the needs of patients, society and the profession. If medicine fails to demonstrate these attributes, it will lose its status as a profession. Thus, professionalism relates to the contract between the medical profession, the individual patient and their family and society.

Challenges to medical professionalism

The practice of medicine has undergone significant change over the years (see also Chapter 4). In the United States, for example, a healthcare insurance system was instituted, which has evolved into one that is seen as inefficient and unable to provide for the basic medical needs of Americans. The second half of the twentieth century was marked also by the development of a variety of unified national systems in developed countries. There have been innovative scientific discoveries including major pharmacological breakthroughs, completion of the genome project and the rapid advancement of molecular genetics. Computer technology and clinical information systems have affected many practice management functions. However, economic constraints have impacted the amount of time physicians spend with patients. Americans are concerned about the high costs of medical care and the rate of medical errors. Additional regulations on physician practices are viewed as constraints, and many physicians feel pressured by the business and political aspects of their work. The ethics of the commercialism that entered into healthcare in many countries, especially from the pharmaceutical industry, is often counter to the ethics of medical professionalism. Physicians have thus been challenged to preserve the doctor–patient relationship and to withstand threats to their professionalism.

In many countries, and certainly in the United States, physicians have felt disenfranchised from the process of resolving these problems, especially by efforts to remove some of the traditional privileges which had been granted to the profession by society. For example, employers and government, concerned about escalating healthcare costs, have introduced new clinical parameters such as managed care. These have impacted the autonomy of physicians in their care to patients (Barondess 2003).

The profession and public trust

The medical profession has historically responded to questions raised about the quality of healthcare and medical education. The American Medical Association, in the early 1900s, founded its Council on Medical Education to strengthen medical education and improve healthcare. As noted by Weissman and Busch in this volume, the resultant Flexner Report of 1910 brought about sweeping changes in medical education around the world, many of which are still in place today (Flexner 1910).

As training in medicine became more formalized, and with the explosion of knowledge, areas of clinical specialization were established. Specialist physicians, concerned about the quality of care and the standards of training, established boards to certify physicians as qualified specialists. The American Board of Medical Specialties (ABMS) was established in 1933 to oversee the standards of specialty boards and for the development of future boards (Brennan *et al.* 2004). The American Board of Psychiatry and Neurology (ABPN) was incorporated the following year (Juul *et al.* 2004).

To maintain public trust and to assure there are qualified physicians to deliver care to the public, the doctors in many countries, including the United States, established accrediting bodies to oversee medical student education and residency training. There are, however, a number of countries which still lack national standards for postgraduate education. In addition, in the United States, specific licensure requirements to practise medicine were established by each state, unlike many countries with national standards. Specialty boards in the United States provided mechanisms for board certification and recertification. A system was developed for continuing medical education to provide updated medical knowledge for those in practice. Hospitals now assess the qualifications of physicians applying for medical staff privileges. These measures provide the public with assurance of a standardized evaluation of medical qualifications, with the implicit promise of high levels of professionalism.

With the dramatic changes in healthcare organization, financing and delivery systems, society's views and expectations of physicians have evolved. In the mid 1990s, leaders in US medical education questioned whether the medical school curriculum adequately prepared students to practise medicine in the complexities of the approaching twenty-first century. The result was an initiative by the Association of American Medical Colleges (AAMC) to review the design and content of medical education. Beginning in 1996, the Medical School Objectives Project (MSOP) developed a set of goals and objectives to guide individual medical school curriculum review. The Project sought broad representation, reviewing input from 14 participating countries as well as from citizen groups and scholars. The result was the identification of four professional attributes that physicians must possess at the completion of their training to meet the changing needs of society. The four attributes are altruism, knowledge, skill and duty (AAMC 1998). The Project identified learning objectives for each attribute to be used as a reference for further curriculum assessment. The MSOP report encouraged the development of outcome measures for each of the objectives. Although professionalism was not specifically identified, all four components addressed many values identified with professionalism.

In 1999, the US Institute of Medicine (IOM) issued a report on medical errors and deaths (IOM 1999). This brought public attention to the need for safety and quality improvement in the healthcare system. The IOM report expressed concern that inadequate physician training in the United States might contribute to the poor quality of care. Because our profession has the responsibility to monitor its education and training standards and to assure the competence of its practitioners, the IOM asserted that individual physicians have a responsibility to society and to themselves to maintain their expertise.

Prior to the IOM report, the US Department of Education mandated outcome measures for all educational programmes receiving federal funding. It would no longer be acceptable to report what students were to be taught, but rather to demonstrate proficiency on outcome evaluations. Focus was placed on medical education because of its heavy public funding. The Accreditation Council for Graduate Medical Education (ACGME), the US accrediting agency which establishes national standards for residency and fellowship training in various medical specialties, began to develop measurable objectives to assess outcomes in physician training. Parallel initiatives have occurred in many areas of the world, for example in the Union of European Medical Specialists (UEMS), although legal implications may well vary.

Concurrently the ABMS, the umbrella organization of 24 medical specialty boards, was also working on outcome measures for the evaluation and certification of physician specialists. Board certification provides assurance to the public that such specialists have successfully completed an approved education and residency training, have obtained licensure and have passed an evaluative process to assess their ability to provide quality care in that specialty.

In 1999, the ACGME and ABMS jointly delineated six core competency categories for all physicians, thus establishing what could become a continuum of medical education, certification and lifelong physician development. These are patient care, medical knowledge, interpersonal and communication skills, practice-based learning and improvement, professionalism and systems-based practice. Competency in patient care includes that which is compassionate, appropriate and effective for the treatment of health problems and the promotion of health. The medical knowledge competency is about established and evolving biomedical, clinical and cognate (such as epidemiological and socio-behavioural) sciences and the application of this knowledge to patient care. The interpersonal and communication skills result in effective information exchange and teaming with patients, their families and other health professionals. Competency in practice-based learning and improvement involves investigation and evaluation of patient care, appraisal and assimilation of scientific evidence and improvements in patient care based on self-evaluation and lifelong learning. Professionalism is demonstrated by a commitment to carrying out professional responsibilities, adherence to ethical principles and sensitivity to a diverse patient population. Systems-based practice is manifested by an awareness of and responsiveness to the larger context and system for healthcare, and the ability to effectively call on system resources to provide optimum healthcare (ACGME Outcome Project 2006). It is clear that all components define the linkage of expertise and professionalism.

The ACGME mandated the implementation of training in all core competencies. Since 1 July 2002, each accredited residency programme in the United States has been required to teach and assess trainees in these competencies and in specialty-specific competencies (e.g. the ability to carry out a suicide risk assessment). The ABMS determined that its specialty boards should utilize relevant core competencies in each of the six areas in specialty and subspecialty evaluations for the initial certification process and in the maintenance of certification (Batalden *et al.* 2002, ABMS Maintenance of Certification 2009). These efforts have changed the way US medicine has viewed graduate medical education and professional development, as a lifelong process linking expertise to professionalism.

Competencies in medical education

The significance of the movement towards competency-based medical student and residency education should not be minimized. In competency-based medical education, the focus is on the trainee's performance towards achieving the goals and objectives of the curriculum, not on the assessment of the content of the curriculum. The performance or educational outcome is evaluated to ensure completion of the learning objective. Competency-based education requires written goals and objectives for each learning experience and a variety of assessment methods to measure the resident's learning outcome. For example, a resident assigned to an inpatient psychiatry rotation has goals and objectives related to conducting a comprehensive interview during a new patient admission. The resident's interview skill, for example, would be assessed by direct observation and a review of the admission work-up to determine if the objectives of the learning experience were met. End-of-rotation global assessments would no longer be adequate because they fail to address the individual learning outcomes met on the rotation. An extensive description of competency-based education and evaluation can be found on the ACGME website.

The goal of the ACGME outcome project is to establish a framework for residents to develop competence as a physician. A second goal is to improve patient care by improving the quality of resident education and training. A physician who has successfully met competencies will possess medical knowledge, render quality patient care, demonstrate professionalism, utilize good interpersonal and communication skills, understand the importance of systems-based practice, be able to critically evaluate the literature and use self-reflection to evaluate their own practice, including the need for improvement. Although in this paradigm professionalism is defined as a specific competency, one could argue that all six areas relate to components of professionalism.

The ACGME, through its specialty-specific residency review committees, monitors programme adherence in every accredited postgraduate programme in the United States. The committees assess training requirements while focusing on evidence that programmes are making data-driven improvements in resident performance and outcome measures. The implementation process is still ongoing, although much progress has been made.

While the ACGME utilizes the 'threshold' model of competency measure for residents in training (i.e. the resident either has the competency or does not), the ACGME does support the educational philosophy that physicians acquire competencies throughout their professional development (Leach 2002). This is consistent with the belief of the Accreditation Council for Continued Medical Education (ACCME), which is responsible for the continuing medical education of practising physicians as part of their learning process towards expertise (Heffron *et al.* 2007).

A way to view lifelong learning and competency development is to utilize the Dreyfus model of knowledge acquisition. Commissioned by the US Air Force to understand the skill development of air force pilots, Dreyfus and Dreyfus described five stages of knowledge development: novice, advanced beginner, competent, proficient and expert. These stages of learning have also been applied to other professional endeavours. The Dreyfus model describes the mental processing, logic, rules and principles that guide reasoning as one advances through the various stages of skill attainment (Dreyfus and Dreyfus 1986).

For example, a novice medical student uses rule-oriented behaviour and memorization to begin learning medicine. The advanced beginner, in the third and fourth year of medical school, notes the recurrent meaning of situations seen in clinical work and begins to use rules and principles to guide learning. During residency, the competent trainee can plan, organize and prioritize work. Residents understand the risks and consequences of their actions, which provide opportunities for study and reflection in learning. A proficient physician who has completed residency continues to hone skills in assessment and efficiency, while developing a holistic sense of practice. The expert physician has an intuitive grasp on what should occur, is attuned to subtle changes in expected patterns and knows how to make corrections (Batalden *et al.* 2002).

On the completion of residency, graduates should have achieved competence in the six ACGME core competencies as an entry-level physician. Certifying boards are now developing processes to evaluate these competencies at the initial certification and in the maintenance of certification. This will provide for a seamless, continuous process towards maintaining expertise and professionalism.

Competency-based efforts are also being used as a framework for continuing medical education for practising physicians. The ACCME, a major accrediting body for institutions and organizations offering continuing medical education, established new guidelines for continuing medical education in the United States in 2003 after convening a Task Force on Competency and Continuum of Medical Education. These guidelines support the professional development of physicians by recommending continuous improvement in knowledge and practice performance (Regnier *et al.* 2005). The UEMS has a similar process. The ACCME has endorsed the identification of common terms and definitions so that competency expectations are shared across the continuum of medical education. The third report on quality of healthcare produced by the IOM recommended five competencies that health professions must incorporate into all educational curricula. These are in harmony with those of the ACGME-ABMS utilized for the accreditation of graduate medical education programmes and the maintenance of certification programmes for board-certified physicians in the United States. The ACCME model of continuing professional development embraces these competencies and stresses lifelong learning, self-assessment and evaluation of performance in practice with learning activities that update skills.

Although graduate medical education through the ACGME was the first to fully implement competency-based education, US medical schools also have competency goals in their curriculum. The Liaison Committee on Medical Education (LCME) is the accrediting body for US medical schools (LCME 2009). Accreditation by the LCME is required for schools to receive federal grants and to participate in federal loan programmes. Most state boards of medical licensure require that US medical schools be LCME accredited as a condition for licensure of their graduates. The United States Medical Licensing Examination (USMLE) programme requires a three-part assessment of medical trainees as a prerequisite to medical licensure. US medical students must be enrolled in an LCME-accredited school to take the exams. Also, to be eligible for an ACGME-accredited residency programme, applicants must be graduates of an LCME-accredited school. Institutional accreditation by the LCME assures that medical education encompasses standardized learning experiences and academic endeavours. Thus, LCME accreditation fosters quality teaching and institutional and programme improvement.

The LCME has accreditation standards for education which addresses competencies. For LCME accreditation, the written objectives of the educational programme must be structured in outcome-based terms that allow assessment of medical student competencies. These outcome measures must reflect how well graduates of the programme develop competencies in knowledge, skills, attitudes and the values necessary for a residency. This links expertise and professionalism early in medical training. Each medical school is required to define the professional attributes it adopts on the basis of the school's mission and the community in which it exists, allowing for flexibility based on local values and culture. The LCME recognizes the professional attributes of a physician, including those identified by the AAMC Medical School Objectives Project, the competencies of the ACGME-ABMS and the physician roles summarized in the 2000 CanMEDS report (Royal College of Physicians and Surgeons of Canada 1996).

Competencies in certification

When board certification in the United States was first established to quantify and qualify the knowledge and skills of specialty physicians, the certification was an official recognition that was valid for life. Board certification has required successful performance on a proctored cognitive examination. Some specialty boards have also required oral examinations, audits of records or case logs or observed performance with patients or standardized patients. Board certification has been viewed as one of the most important professional qualifications for physicians and is recognized and highly valued by the public when seeking a qualified phys–ician. People generally believe that a board-certified physician provides a higher quality of healthcare (Brennan *et al.* 2004). Although this is voluntary, most physicians in the United States seek certification in their specialty. The rate of expansion of scientific discoveries and medical knowledge, however, has led to concern that some who have obtained past board certification may not be staying current in their field. Arguments were made for time-limited certificates as early as 1940, but the first time-limited certificate was not issued until 1970 by the American Board of Family Practice, now Family Medicine (Rhodes 2007). The ABPN began issuing time-limited certification on 1 October 1994. All board certifications by the

ABPN are now valid for a 10-year period. Physicians who received board certification before the 1994 change are exempted from recertification.

Physicians with time-limited certificates must complete a recertification process within the time frame specified by their specialty board. Examinations assess the knowledge and qualifications of physicians at the time of the recertification but do not provide evidence of their actual practice.

A recent systematic review in the United States of the relationship between clinical experience and quality of healthcare found that physicians who have been in practice longer may have a decline in practice performance and patient outcomes (Choudry *et al.* 2005). Of course, satisfactory performance on one recertification examination does not guarantee competence in practice. In response to this and other issues, in 2000 the ABMS mandated that all physicians with time-limited certificates participate in a Maintenance of Certification (MOC) programme to retain their board certification. MOC requires documentation of continuous professional development, with the goal of ensuring continued competence of board-certified practising physicians. MOC requires the physician to be an active participant in the learning process and to give feedback on what was learnt. The philosophy embodied here is that improvement in practice requires assessment. The ABMS requires that all member boards incorporate the six core competencies into a four-part MOC framework. The physician must demonstrate evidence of: (1) professional standing by possessing a valid, unrestricted medical licence; (2) lifelong learning and self-assessment; (3) cognitive expertise demonstrated by a standardized examination; and (4) practice performance assessment compared with peers and national benchmarks, with improvement recommendations and follow-up assessments (Brennan *et al.* 2004). Each ABMS board was mandated to design specific methods for its specialty members to ensure continuous MOC.

In response to the MOC mandate, the ABPN established a Core Competency Committee, which developed the infrastructure for the ongoing review and validation of core psychiatric and neurological competencies. They determined which competencies would be assessed at the initial certification and which would be assessed by the ABPN-MOC programme. Although there were some common core competencies for psychiatry and neurology, each of them had its own specialty-specific core competencies. The psychiatry core competencies were approved by the ABPN in January 2003 (Scheiber *et al.* 2003). The ABMS has charged the ABPN with ensuring that each of the relevant core competencies is assessed at least once during its MOC cycle. At present, the MOC programme for US psychiatrists requires proof of licensure, a cognitive examination and evidence of lifelong learning and self-assessment. There is a phase-in period for the requirement to demonstrate practice assessment with practice improvement efforts. Once implemented in 2013, this module will assess competency in professionalism and communication by requiring that physicians provide patient and peer feedback concerning their clinical practice (Juul 2004).

Competencies in licensure and credentialing

A competency framework is being used by organizations that grant medical licensure and credentialing. The US Federation of State Medical Boards (FSMB) is the parent organization composed of 70 state medical boards in the United States and its territories (AMA 2009, Federation of State Medical Boards 2009). It works with state medical boards to improve healthcare by promoting high standards for physician licensure and practice. Each state medical board shares in the responsibility to protect the public through the regulation of physicians and other healthcare providers. Each board has the authority to license physicians, regulate the practice of medicine and discipline those who violate the medical practice standards of the state.

Physicians seeking licensure in the United States and its territories must apply to the state medical licensing authority. The licence to practise medicine is granted by the state authority only after verification of qualifications for licensure. The FSMB, in collaboration with the National Board of Medical Examiners (NBME), provides two programmes for use by state medical licensing boards on which to base their decision. The first is the USMLE exam programme, and the second is the Post-Licensure Assessment System (PLAS).

The USMLE programme provides a three-step process for initial licensure of all graduates of LCME-accredited medical schools in the United States and Canada, and all international medical graduates seeking residency training and medical licensure in the United States. Graduates of accredited US osteopathic medical schools can either choose the USMLE or they may also meet state licensure requirements through completion of the osteopathic licensure process. The primary purpose of the USMLE is to provide information to state medical licensing boards by assessing the competencies of physicians applying for licensure. The USMLE recently reviewed the design and test format to ensure the examination process measured the competencies required by the profession. It recommended a revision of the USMLE to include competencies using a model consistent with national standards, such as those identified by the ACGME (Comprehensive Review of USMLE 2008). The PLAS provides services to medical licensing authorities utilizing assessments to measure the competence of licensed physicians or previously licensed physicians who are seeking re-registration.

Although not yet mandated by all US state licensing boards, most states require participation in continuing medical education as part of the licence renewal process. Board certification and MOC programmes require an unrestricted medical licence as well as evidence of continuing medical education. Thus, competency-based education and physician assessments have become a seamless process from medical student education through to residency, licensure, board certification and MOC.

In 2004, the FSMB adopted a policy statement reaffirming the state medical board's responsibility to ensure the competence of physicians seeking relicensure. However, because each state licensing board operates under its own state statute, new legislation, passed on a state-by-state basis, would be necessary to change the requirements for licensure or relicensure (Steinbrook 2005). The FBMS is continuing work on a Maintenance of Licensure (MOL) initiative and has adopted principles to guide further policy development in this area.

Physician competence and professionalism are also reviewed as part of credentialing and public accountability (Cassel and Holmboe 2006). Hospital credentialing is required by the US Joint Commission on Accreditation of Healthcare Organizations standards for accreditation. The Joint Commission, formerly referred to as JCAHO, is an organization that evaluates and accredits over 15 000 healthcare organizations and programmes in the United States according to performance standards for safe, high-quality care (AMA 2009). In addition, US insurance panels require verification of physician qualifications (Amerongen 2002).

Both hospitals and health plan panels review board certification and MOC data, but some do not require board certification for credentialing. The Joint Commission requires that hospitals develop a credible process to determine competency of physicians providing clinical care to patients in the hospital. The credentialing and privileging processes involve evaluation of physician performance along the six areas of ACGME-ABMS competencies. Hospital privileging decisions are made by medical staff committees and approved by members of a governing body. Although it is difficult to assess the professionalism and expertise of individual doctors who are credentialed by a review of licensure, education, training and current clinical competence, the integration of the core competencies into the credentialing standards attempts to provide a comprehensive evaluation that links expertise and professionalism in actual practice.

For Joint Commission accreditation status, which provides the public with a measure of quality and safe patient care, hospitals must have medical staff rules for self-governance and a process to ensure ongoing quality of its physicians. They also recommend that hospitals develop ways to address lack of professionalism on the part of the medical staff. This includes disciplinary actions such as loss of clinical privileges and reports to professional licensure bodies.

As physicians are required to present outcome data for ongoing documentation of their performance, both hospitals and insurance health plans have the potential to provide physicians with relevant information about patients whom they have cared for within those systems. This would serve to reduce redundancy of data collection and a mechanism to provide the same data to numerous requesting agencies and organizations (Cassel and Holmboe 2006).

Conclusions

Expertise and medical professionalism are inextricably linked. The field of medicine has a duty and a responsibility to society, our patients and the profession to ensure the continuous expertise and professionalism of its members. These characteristics of clinical excellence are being assessed more closely as part of the profession's public accountability. To carry out this task, educational institutions, professional organizations and societies, licensing boards and accrediting agencies have been called upon to develop interlocking and overlapping systems to monitor and assess the presence of these qualities throughout the field.

The process of utilizing competencies as a framework for assessing expertise and professionalism is in continuous development. There are still many unanswered questions, therefore, about how to provide useful information about physician competence and professionalism to the public. In addition, physicians will need to address how best to monitor the competence of non-board-certified colleagues, those with lifelong board certification and those who are not in clinical practice but continue to hold an active medical licence.

In the past 50 years, many countries have established unified national health systems of care that differ from the historical model of medicine, which emphasized much more independent, individual decision-making about practice. An important question regarding the shift in systems of care is how physician values have been impacted by this change in practice. This could be accomplished by an evaluation of professionalism among physicians to assess if and how each system of healthcare influences professional behaviours.

Physicians and the public understand the linkage between expertise and medical professionalism, but both groups are still working to clarify the best ways to foster these qualities and to assess their presence in clinicians. The role of continuing medical education following completion of formal training has evolved as one way to encourage continuing expertise, and most countries now have requirements for the ongoing assessment of continuing education efforts. The view that medical education is a lifelong learning progression towards physician expertise is a paradigm shift for some, but it is one which the field has agreed does indeed benefit both the patient and the physician.

References

ACGME Outcome Project (2006). www.acgme. org/Outcome/. Last accessed 9 September 2009.

American Board of Medical Specialties (2009). *Maintenance of Certification*. http://abms. org/Maintenance_of_Certification/. Last accessed 9 September 2009.

American Medical Association (2009). *State Medical Licensure Requirements and Statistics*. Chicago: AMA.

Amerongen D (2002). Physician credentialing in a consumer-centric world. *Health Tracking* **21**, 152–156.

Association of American Medical Colleges (1998). *Medical School Objectives Project Report I: Learning Objectives for Medical Student Education*. www.AAMC.org. Last accessed 9 September 2009.

Barondess J A (2003). Medicine and professionalism. *Archives of Internal Medicine* **163**, 145–149.

Batalden P, Leach D, Swing S, Dreyfus H, Dreyfus S (2002). General competencies and accreditation in graduate medical education. *Health Affairs* **21**, 103–111.

Brennan T, Horwitz R, Duffy F D, Cassel C, Goode L, Lipner R (2004). The role of physician specialty board certification status in the quality movement. *Journal of the American Medical Association* **292**, 1038–1043.

Cassel C, Holmboe E (2006). Credentialing and public accountability. *Journal of the American Medical Association* **295**, 939–940.

Choudry N K, Fletcher R H, Soumerai S B (2005). Systemic review: the relationship between clinical experience and the quality of health care. *Annals of Internal Medicine* **142**, 260–273.

Cohen J D (2006). Professionalism in medical education, an American perspective: from evidence to accountability. *Medical Education* **40**, 607–617.

Comprehensive Review of USMLE. CEUP Summary of the Final Report and Recommendations (2008). www.usmle.org/general_information/CEUP-Summary-Report-June2008.pdf. Last accessed 9 September 2009.

Dreyfus H, Dreyfus S (1986). *Mind over Machine*. New York: Free Press.

Federation of State Medical Boards (2009). www.fsmb.org. Last accessed 9 September 2009.

Flexner A (1910). *Medical Education in the United States and Canada*. Boston: Merrymount Press.

Heffron M G, Simspon D, Kochar M S (2007). Competency-based physician education, recertification, and licensure. *Wisconsin Medical Journal* **106**, 215–218.

L T Kohn, J M Corrigan, M S Donaldson (eds.) and the Institute of Medicine (1999). *To Err Is Human: Building a Safer Health System*. Washington, DC: National Academy Press.

Juul D, Scheiber SC, Kramer TA (2004). Subspecialty certification by the American Board of Psychiatry and Neurology. *Academic Psychiatry* **28**, 12–17.

Lathan S R (2002). Medical professionalism: a parsonian view. *The Mount Sinai Journal of Medicine* **69**, 363–369.

Leach D (2002). Competence is habit. *Journal of the American Medical Association* **287**, 243–244.

Liaison Committee on Medical Education (2009). *Overview: Accreditation and the LCME*. www.LCME.org. Last accessed 9 September 2009.

MacKenzie C R (2007). Professionalism and medicine. *Hospital for Special Surgery Journal* **3**, 222–227.

Regnier K, Kopelow M, Lane D, Alden E (2005). Accreditation for learning and change: quality and improvement as the outcome. *The Journal of Continuing Education in the Health Professions* **25**, 174–182.

Rhodes R S (2007). Maintenance of certification. *The American Surgeon* **73**, 143–147.

Royal College of Physicians and Surgeons of Canada (1996). *CanMEDS 2000 Project Report*. Ottawa: The Royal College of Physicians and Surgeons of Canada.

Scheiber S C, Kramer T A, Adamowski S E (2003). The implications of core competencies for psychiatric education and practice in the US. *Canadian Journal of Psychiatry* **48**, 215–220.

Steinbrook R (2005). Renewing board certification. *New England Journal of Medicine* **353**, 1994–1997.

Stern D (2006). *Measuring Medical Professionalism*. New York: Oxford University Press.

Swick H M (2000). Toward a normative definition of medical professionalism. *Academic Medicine* **75**, 612–616.

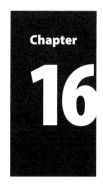

Chapter

16

Leadership and professionalism

Helen Herrman, Julian Freidin and Sharon Brownie

Editors' introduction

Leadership is a core component of medical professionalism. The leadership here is not necessarily related to being a clinical leader, but to providing a role which allows the clinician to take an overview of the service, thereby planning service delivery and service development. This role focuses on horizon scanning and thinking ahead to deal with potential threats and looming changes. Leadership in multidisciplinary teams is one example of leadership, but the role of the psychiatrist in taking the lead on developing and delivering public mental health agendas is equally distinct and valid. Herrman *et al.* start from this very point and argue that there must be a distinction between these roles and the leadership role related to policy-making. Contemporary ideas of leadership in mental health are related to international methods of healthcare and collaborative practice. The latter includes patient (consumer) focus, mutual respect, shared understanding, clarification of functions and roles, along with increased efficiency and effectiveness. There has to be a move away from charismatic leadership to a more distributed model of leadership. Links with local stakeholders, communication abilities and the aptitude to empower others are all important leadership skills. Leaders can not only support professionalism within the practice context, they can also provide joint working. The role of the leader in clinical teams is collaborative. Training individuals in such skills, along with preparing them for a broader public mental health agenda, is an investment worth making. In addition, collaborating with other sectors such as education, primary care, employment, the justice system, etc. should form an integral part of the role of the leader. Leadership by the professional societies in areas of mental health policy development and the interface with governments and policy-makers should also be key external roles that will allow the societies to remain relevant in the contemporary world whilst internally supporting their members in developing broad-based portfolios to deliver high-quality services.

Introduction

Psychiatrists and other mental health professionals who work in clinical care, service management or policy development have various understandings about leadership. When these understandings are challenged, lack of clarity and possible conflict about leadership can undermine effectiveness and challenge professional identity. Examining ideas about leadership in mental health can help professionals to work more effectively and with more satisfaction.

Professionalism in Mental Healthcare: Experts, Expertise and Expectations, ed. Dinesh Bhugra and Amit Malik. Published by Cambridge University Press. © Cambridge University Press 2011.

Today's mental health professionals face new leadership concepts, two of which, while offering the possibility of improved practice, pose significant challenges. The first challenge relates to the increasingly common practice of mental health professionals working together in teams, in collaborative clinical care. In many countries it is unusual for mental health-care to be provided by a single professional even when one person is designated as the main direct-care provider. However, new collaborative care approaches engender new ideas about leadership and encourage psychiatrists, for example, to clarify what forms of leadership are required and how to become competent in these. Contemporary thinking suggests that they need to position themselves as leaders who can work effectively in partnership with others in their community to improve mental health.

The second type of challenge arises from the broader development in public policy and health policy of partnerships between service providers and the need for new forms of distributed leadership. In complex settings of this kind, professional competence requires an individual to interact in new ways so as to exert appropriate authority and provide leadership of various kinds without necessarily being the organizational leader.

Professional bodies working together can help to define the distinction between professionalism and the leadership of teams, services or policy-making. This chapter examines the concepts of leadership within contemporary practice and policy contexts. Discussion focuses on the range of ways that mental health professionals can lead and participate in promoting mental health with the engagement of clinical team members, professional organizations, employers and policy-makers.

Contemporary ideas about leadership in mental healthcare

Over the past two decades, public policy-makers have introduced models of joint and collaborative working with the aim of improving social and economic outcomes (Considine 1994, Morgan 1997, Considine 2004, OECD 2006). This is a complex and continually evolving public policy development evident in a broad range of contexts, including health services (Jackson *et al.* 2006, Stone 2007).

International public health policy has seen a dramatic shift from isolated models of healthcare towards 'new governance' healthcare arrangements that support local health systems responsible for the health needs of a community (Lomas *et al.* 1997, Jackson *et al.* 2006). This trend towards inter-agency collaboration is evident at the clinical level, where the increasing complexity of healthcare has generated an expectation and a need for health professionals from various disciplines to work as a team. Often referred to as the 'new professionalism', the expectation for clinicians is to participate in a shift in clinical practice towards collaborative models of care.The shift in practice is supported by growing evidence that effective interdisciplinary practice improves consumer health outcomes (Stone 2007). The main idea behind these public policy trends is that interorganizational and interdisciplinary collaboration in service delivery is more effective than systems that lack a focus on such a collaboration; that is, if everyone co-operates, improved results will be achieved (D'amour *et al.* 2005, OECD 2006, Brownie 2007).

Along with the shift in practice, there is recognition that effective collaborative practice doesn't 'just happen' (Craven and Bland 2006). Health systems in high- and middle-income countries worldwide are seeking to define the best ways to promote and support collaborative practice (Hall 2005). The development of effective collaborative practice requires complex strategies that address structural factors (systems, tools) and human relationships at a local level (Horby 1993, Craven and Bland 2006). Effective networks can help to identify and lower systemic barriers to collaboration. For example, referral protocols can improve communication between primary and secondary care and encourage the development of productive working relationships between service providers.

In mental healthcare, there are several important elements of collaborative care. These include a consumer focus, mutual respect, shared understanding about the purpose of mental healthcare, clarification of functions and roles and increased efficiency and effectiveness, as well as integration or partnerships between generalist and specialist service providers and a view of primary care as part of a wider system of health and social care (Brewis and Hurford 2004).

How, then, is leadership defined within this increasingly collaborative context? Although the terms 'leader' and 'leadership' are much used, they are poorly understood (Hosking 1988), despite evidence of studies about leadership and leadership characteristics that can be traced back over several centuries (Higgs 2002). In 2000, Coffee and Jones estimated that more than 2000 books were published on the topic of leadership. By 2002, Aitken discovered more than 8000 works in a search of the Library of Congress database. The special edition on leadership in the *Harvard Business Review* in December 2001 is testimony to the enduring fascination with the topic (Higgs 2002). This discussion is focused on leadership in the context of partnership-based collaborative care.

Leadership – it is a set of focus-enhancing or unity-enhancing behaviours that help some collectivity … accomplish useful work. (Bardach 1998, p. 223)

Leadership is identified as a specific variable affecting the quality of outcomes and is associated with the enactment of the 'new professionalism', a central element in successfully adopting partnership-based policy and collaborative care. The attitude and behaviour of clinicians, including their willingness or otherwise to accept leadership responsibilities, have a significant effect on success or failure in establishing effective service systems (Newton 2009).

Grint (1997) describes how traditional concepts of leadership are based on trait and situational and contingency approaches, and new ideas about leadership are emerging in contemporary contexts (Greenleaf 1977, Spears 1995, Grint 1997, Bardach 1998, Yukl 1998, Wheatley 1999, Frydman *et al.* 2000). Given the complexity of networked local development and interorganizational partnerships in many contemporary systems, Starr (2001) describes a distributed theory of leadership. Leaders exist at many levels within a network. In such settings, effective leadership is distributed or stretched across two or more of these leaders, who may work independently in either the same or separate organizations. They share common aspirations, goals and objectives. If the leaders' efforts become complementary, the whole may be greater than the sum of the parts.

Sergiovanni defines community as 'a collection of individuals who are … bound to shared ideas and ideals' (Sergiovanni 1994, p. 218). A community of clinicians is bound together accordingly by a set of collectively shared values (Newton 2009). An effective collaborative team is made up of a community of people associating and networked together, with a common purpose. Such contexts appear to require leaders who have a ' … transformative and/or facilitative style, and distribute leadership throughout the system' (Starr 2001, p. 13).

To help to achieve common goals, interorganizational partnerships often establish various steering structures such as joint forums, boards or councils, implementation networks or project teams. Bardach (1998) believes that leadership can help to diagnose problems, introduce improvements in the interorganizational system and subsystems, engender trust between key players, secure resources, agree short- and long-term strategies and reduce barriers to success. His functional definition of leadership for interorganizational contexts (above) does not offer comment about a particular setting, about who will perform the leadership activities and what style the leadership behaviours may take. Nor does it imply that the leadership behaviours belong to any particular individual; they could be performed by any number of individuals distributed within the interorganizational system or subsystem. Consequently, leadership is noted as a shared activity. Synonymous with these concepts is that of power sharing, which DuBrin and Dalglish (2003) regard as an important feature of newly emerging leadership models. These concepts are congruent with that of distributed leadership across a complex system and subsystems of networks and associations. Just as the collaborative network forms a system, leadership too can be viewed as a system of supporting and complementary behaviours helping the collaborative achieve its goals.

Within a distributed leadership system, the 'key individuals' or 'charismatic policy drivers' seen as central to the success of the sustainable local development agenda are not necessarily the individuals with the obvious pre-existing legitimate authority. The leaders that emerge, however, have capacity to 'drive the process forward', along with the commitment, skills and charisma to motivate others (Evans *et al.* 2005, p. 110). Rather than being formally appointed, the leaders may emerge from a variety of points as the incentives and benefits of collaboration become clearer. This then has a flow-on effect, as these visionary individuals, with enthusiasm and a vision of how to solve problems and make progress, mobilize others to participate (Chrislip 2002).

The style fits with the notion of servant leadership that Greenleaf first mooted in 1977, whereby individuals – of any station in life – act through excellence and with the intent to build a better society. Spears (1995) acknowledges Greenleaf's notion of servant leadership, arguing that it has influenced many contemporary management thinkers.

The leadership concepts of 'key individuals', 'charismatic policy drivers' and 'servant leaders' that Greenleaf (1977) coined, should not be confused with the frequently reinforced notion of heroic leaders (Frydman *et al.* 2000). Sustainable collaboration requires leaders who can enable teams to face and resolve common problems. Chrislip (2002, p.17) believes that '…heroic leadership cannot enhance the civic community because it denies, fundamentally, the notion of shared responsibility.'

Modern leadership descriptors include leadership characteristics such as knowledge of and connectedness with the local context and the external environment, communication and empowerment of others, an openness to learning even while possessing extraordinary gifts for vision and for strategy, a collaborative rather than competitive approach, ability to bring others together in a constructive manner and a strong commitment to encouraging and supporting others to learn (Senge 1995, Spears 1995, Yukl 1998, Frydman *et al.* 2000, Chrislip 2002). In a clinical context, leaders must have credibility and the capacity to bridge the divides between sectors, cultures and ideologies (Chrislip 2002).

Appropriate leadership is critical to supporting professionalism within current practice settings of increasing networking and joint working. Clear ideas about leadership and its relationship to professionalism are important in the establishment of collaborations and associations of various types in a service system. Good understanding of leadership is critical to the successful implementation of collaborative practice.

Leadership in clinical teams

The way that mental health professionals and others work together has an impact on standards of clinical care and professional satisfaction. In all countries, primary healthcare workers are important participants in care, together with families and consumers. In some high-income countries such as Australia and New Zealand, state-funded mental health services are provided by multidisciplinary teams. In all these settings, effective collaboration and teamwork require agreed goals, an agreed approach, effective communication styles, established ground rules, clear roles and competent leadership (Herrman *et al*. 2002). Collaboration with consumers and families or other carers is an important guide and motivation to finding ways to make this succeed. Effective partnerships with consumers and carers require clinical service providers to commit to listening and responding to the views of the users of their services. Interdisciplinary teamwork can change fundamentally when it becomes apparent, for instance, that a focus on the work done specifically by each profession or the needs of networking are given more attention than acting directly for the benefit of consumers and carers (Macdonald *et al*. 2002).

As described in other chapters, the training of mental health professionals needs to equip them with the attitudes, skills and knowledge to work effectively with others and in multidisciplinary teams. This requires professional associations to develop appropriate educational aims and objectives for trainees and supervisors. Through the Royal Australian and New Zealand College of Psychiatrists, for example, training in teamwork is accomplished through workplace supervision and didactic teaching, and the results are assessed by supervisors as well as by formal examination (Burke *et al*. 2000). Ideally, in any country or community the professional associations for a range of mental health professionals – including psychiatrists, psychologists, nurses, social workers and occupational therapists, as well as primary care doctors – will collaborate or consult with each other and with consumers and carers to design complementary approaches to training and continuing practice.

Leadership in public mental health

Services for people living with mental illnesses have a history of separation from other sectors of healthcare and community life. This has had deleterious effects on the care and welfare of those with illnesses, as well as on the mental health of the population. It contributes to separation between the policy-makers and planners in mental health and those in primary care and other health services, and in public health. However, awareness is growing that mental health is part of health and that mental health is promoted through population-based public health measures, as well as health system change (Herrman *et al*. 2005, Barry and Jenkins 2007, Friedli and Parsonage 2007). As part of their contemporary professional role, mental health professionals are often well placed to raise awareness about the possibilities and effectiveness of promoting mental health through the work of other sectors, as well as through health services.

Collaboration of mental health professionals with other sectors

In all countries, mental health professionals have a number of roles in promoting population mental health. They can be advocates for population mental health, technical advisers on health promotion and prevention programme development, leaders or collaborators in such programmes, researchers and professional care providers (Saxena *et al*. 2006). To do this work they need good communication with policy-makers and other professionals and with the general population. They can advise public health planners and programme developers on the effective interventions possible in a number of community sectors (Herrman *et al*.

2005, Barry and Jenkins 2007). They can also work in various partnership roles with primary healthcare.

In *primary healthcare*, mental health professionals can liaise with workers, planners and policy-makers about interventions at individual, service or community levels. Specific initiatives include support for the psychosocial management of communicable and non-communicable diseases, the mental health of mothers, mentally healthy aging, suicide prevention, the physical health of people living with mental illnesses and brief interventions for tobacco smoking and the harmful use of alcohol.

In *schools and the education sector*, mental health professionals provide advice on several types of interventions. Universal school mental health promotion and long-term interventions involving changes to school climate are recognized as effective mental health promotion strategies. Other interventions include the introduction of life skills training aiming to increase social and emotional competence and positive behaviours among pupils, and targeted programmes and clinical services – including group and individual counselling – that aim to increase resilience in children and adolescents who are struggling with stressful life events such as death of a family member or parental divorce, social isolation or immigration status. All of these programmes can benefit in different ways from the collaboration of mental health professionals with school authorities. Mental health professionals working with schools can, among other things, advocate on behalf of children and families to obtain access to needed community resources.

In the *employment, labour and work sector*, mental health professionals can support counselling or job search training for unemployed people living with depression to help them to cope with unemployment and reduce the negative effects on mental health. In the *community sector*, prenatal and infancy home visiting programmes and other support for psychosocial stimulation of infants are important means of population-wide support for early child development and mental health, especially for disadvantaged groups. Mental health professionals can collaborate with primary healthcare workers to give technical advice and training and supervision for the home visitors, who may have a range of backgrounds.

In the *criminal justice system*, persons in custody are a high-risk group for mental illnesses and suicide for several reasons. These include the over-representation of vulnerable groups such as young males, people with addictions and people with mental illnesses, and the major stress of the experience of incarceration. Overworked or untrained correctional staff may miss early warning signs of suicide. Mental health professionals can advise on interventions to improve the mental health status and behaviour of prisoners and minimize the risks of suicide, especially through training and support for correctional staff.

Clinicians and managers in mental health services also need to work with primary healthcare and sectors outside health to ensure the basic conditions are available for effective treatment and recovery. People living with mental illnesses require appropriate housing, income and work, meaningful participation in the community, protection from discrimination and access to education.

Supporting the needs of people living with mental illness and their carers

Mental health professionals play a crucial role in supporting family and other informal carers of people living with mental illnesses. Carers are at increased risk of depression and poor mental health, as well as general ill-health, whether they are caring for young people with schizophrenia or elderly people with dementia. Professional support, self-help groups and other policy and community support can help them in giving care. Professionals can actively collaborate with carers and consumers in clinical care and service development and assist reorientation of services and training (Schofield *et al.* 1998, Froggatt *et al.* 2007).

A range of interventions for people living with mental illness require collaborative work. Examples are the prevention and treatment of physical co-morbidity in people living with mental illnesses. Physical and mental health problems frequently co-occur, although the connections between them are widely underestimated (Prince *et al.* 2007). People living with mental illnesses have a higher risk than others in the same community for physical diseases, intentional or unintentional injuries and premature death. Health services are not provided equitably to people with illnesses, and in most places the quality of care for both mental and physical health conditions for these people needs to be improved (Maj 2009). Mental health professionals also need to ensure that people living with mental illnesses receive advice and support with diet, exercise, relaxation, sleeping strategies, the reduction of stress and interventions for addictions.

The introduction or review of legislation is necessary for protecting the rights of people with mental illnesses, who face stigma, discrimination and marginalization in most societies and a heightened probability of violation of their human rights. There is no national mental health legislation in 25% of the world's countries, accounting for nearly 31% of the global population. The existence of mental health legislation does not necessarily guarantee the protection of the human rights of persons with mental disorders, and in some countries mental health legislation contains provisions that lead to the violation of human rights. Mental health professionals can take a lead to ensure that important matters are addressed in legislation. These include substantive provisions for mental health legislation, including the principle of the least restrictive alternative, confidentiality, informed consent, voluntary and involuntary admission and treatment, an independent review body and competency and guardianship. They also include substantive provisions for other legislation affecting the mental health of people living with mental illnesses, including legislative provisions for protecting the rights of people with mental illnesses in housing, employment and social security (WHO 2005).

Professional bodies as leaders in mental health policy

The professional bodies of psychiatrists and other mental health professionals are uniquely placed to participate in the development of mental health policy and shift the public perception of mental illness. Their colleges, associations and societies bring together extensive expertise and capacity to lead collaborative service development and mental health policy. However, to achieve this leadership role requires a shift in the thinking within those professional bodies if they are to understand this as a potential and useful role for both themselves and the community in which they are located.

Historically, the professional bodies have focused on the needs of their members, creating organizations that have roles including collegial fellowship and mutual support, education of doctors to become psychiatrists, continuing professional development, maintenance of professional standards and financial security of the profession. This strategy is essentially inwardly focused, with the organization interested in its own wellbeing, separate from the needs of the community.

More recently, a number of professional bodies have begun to develop a forward-thinking external focus and policy agenda and to establish strategic partnerships with external organizations. This has occurred in a period when decision-makers in many countries have shown an increased interest in the mental health of the population and have understood that psychiatrists alone cannot provide all the clinical services required. Professional bodies that do not adapt to the needs of the community that funds their members risk being marginalized in the political debate and future service developments.

The rationale for adopting this new direction includes the view that it is essential to position the professional organizations and their members as leaders in a range of activities. The organizations need to anticipate changes and initiatives that are likely to affect health service delivery nationally and globally. They need to develop relationships with policy-makers in health and other relevant areas so that the organization is ready to respond positively and influence policy-making effectively (Freidin 2002, Emmerson 2004).

Change in the health sector will continue and will increasingly affect mental health professionals individually and collectively. In this environment, change is not the variable. The variable is whether psychiatrists, for example, are involved in designing, introducing and directing change that will influence the clinical environment and their work. Such involvement is not a given (Patterson 2002). To do this, the professionals need to understand the systems in which they work. They also need to understand the evidence and experience related to health policy options and the costs and benefits associated with such options. Most fundamentally, new partnerships need to be formed between organizations that share concerns about health system developments. While there are opportunities for professionals to be leaders, a leadership role must be justified.

To be successful, psychiatrists and other mental health professionals and their organizations must embed their activities in the legitimate aspirations of the community. It is not sufficient for psychiatrists to complain about change without offering solutions that are supported and understood by the community. Psychiatrists must communicate to the community – through, for instance, consumer and carer organizations – their clinical, ethical and practical concerns about new models of care, retrograde social policy and other emerging changes or missed opportunities that give concern.

Psychiatrists as leaders can develop a broad national policy portfolio that aims to protect and develop a health system which values human life, high standards of medical practice and a well-trained and adequately resourced workforce that provides the health services the community needs. Professional bodies that choose to take a leadership role in mental health policy can develop aims such as the following:

- Their members play a key role in health systems and financing reform, as well as workforce, public health and social policy initiatives
- Decision-makers understand the need for professional, high-quality and humane clinical care supported by models of delivery and financing that are clinically informed
- Policy-makers are aware of the limitations of trying to 'transplant' the health reforms of other countries without being mindful of local community needs
- Sufficient emphasis is given to the importance of clinical and professional imperatives – the human elements that are often, if not invariably, forgotten in health service developments
- The profession's fundamental roles of maintaining clinical standards are supported and enhanced

The process required to meet these and other aims is complex and will vary between countries. However, there are a number of activities that will help the professional body to move towards a leadership role (Freidin 2002, Emmerson 2004):

- Anticipating issues and initiatives which are likely to affect health service delivery and use established networks to impact positively upon health policy developments
- Developing relationships with health and other relevant policy-makers for the purpose of placing the professional body in a position to influence policy-making
- Obtaining funding for, and undertaking projects relevant to, the professional body and the community
- Developing policy documents and encouraging debate about major health topics
- Developing health policy for the purpose of promoting effective health financing and systems development
- Responding to documents from government agencies and other organizations
- Developing a public profile for the professional body as a repository of credible health policy and planning data
- Developing and extending partnerships and alliances with other health and policy agencies
- Communicating and publicizing policy and policy-making processes through preparation of papers for conference presentations and journal publications
- Developing a database of policy- and programme-related material, and
- Assisting individual psychiatrists with their efforts in policy development in a range of settings by providing relevant data, undertaking policy analysis and providing policy process advice.

Case study: Royal Australian and New Zealand College of Psychiatrists

The Royal Australian and New Zealand College of Psychiatrists (RANZCP) is the principal organization representing the medical specialty of psychiatry in Australia and New Zealand and has responsibility for the training, examining and awarding of the qualification of Fellowship to medical practitioners. There are approximately 2900 Fellows of the RANZCP, who account for approximately 85% of all practising psychiatrists in Australia and over 50% of psychiatrists in New Zealand.

By virtue of their specialist training, psychiatrists bring a comprehensive and integrated biological, psychological, social and cultural approach to the diagnosis, assessment, treatment and prevention of psychiatric disorder and mental health problems. Psychiatrists are uniquely placed to integrate aspects of biological health and illness, psychological function and the individual's social and cultural context. They provide clinical leadership and often work in multidisciplinary team settings. This expertise is also relevant to the development and operation of the whole mental health system to serve the needs of people with mental illness.

In 2004, the rationale for a professional body to show policy leadership as outlined above triggered a shift from the College being an internally focused to an externally focused organization wishing to engage with the community in mental health development. This led to the establishment of the College's policy and project unit; the procurement and delivery of a broad range of projects; the development of extensive resources to support the practice of College members, including those seeking membership; the development of resources for consumers and carers (patients and their families); and the embedding of continued, externally focused partnership activity within the College's stated strategic direction (RANZCP 2008).

The College identified a need for leadership in the following areas:

- Mental health workforce needs
- Improved service integration
- Increased accountability, and
- Increased research opportunities.

The approach taken was to lobby government consistently on these issues, mindful of what was useful to the community and not just to the profession.

Workforce

The development of a sustainable and appropriately trained mental health workforce is critical to the provision of quality mental healthcare for consumers and carers. A professional body that argues only for its own discipline is easily dismissed as self-serving. It has been important to identify the specific roles psychiatrists play within the health workforce, while also arguing for an increasingly competent workforce that includes primary care, general practitioners, nurses and others. This was facilitated by developing a partnership organization with the professional bodies representing general practitioners, psychologists and mental health nurses in order to provide consistency of opinion to government.

Service integration

The RANZCP argued that collaborative approaches which integrate service delivery into a seamless system of diagnosis, treatment and community support are urgently required to allow patients to readily move between service system components. This includes other relevant community services needed by patients with severe mental illness and complex needs with their clinical care (e.g. general healthcare, financial support, housing, substance abuse, rehabilitation, etc.). Optimum care cannot be provided without such a system, and people with mental illness slip through the cracks as opportunities for early intervention and effective treatment are lost. Recovery and rehabilitation are consistently identified by consumers as areas of key importance and should be strongly supported.

Increased accountability

The RANZCP argued for the development of rigorous and ongoing monitoring and evaluation of mental health services, which should involve significant consumer and carer consultation.

Increased research opportunities

The RANZCP argued for increased funding for mental health research. The low level of support was limiting the development and uptake of best practice in mental healthcare in the community. The RANZCP also argued that to inform practical policies there should be an emphasis on applied and consumer- and carer-driven research on interventions and the measurement of service outcomes.

Outcome

An important outcome has been to position the College as a valued contributor to the public debate and mental health policy. There have been strong collaborative activities involving other mental health professions and with community organizations. The role of the psychiatrist in the wellbeing of the community has been enhanced and strengthened in parallel with the improvements in mental health awareness and care.

Conclusions

Mental health professionals are committed to improving the mental health of the individuals and communities with which they work and have unique expertise to contribute. In many countries, they now work in teams and in complex service settings where ideas about leadership are changing. Professionalism needs to be reconciled with distributed leadership and the many roles of mental health professionals. Most professionals are now working in partnerships to support people living with mental illnesses and promote mental health in the community. Professional bodies can make an important contribution to the advancement of mental health and its integration with other health and community sectors; they can achieve this through supporting the changes in orientation of their members and seeking new partnerships to support their own leadership roles in developing health policy and collaboration between sectors and with service users and their families.

References

Aitken P (2002). Introduction to Leadership. Presentation for MDC, Wellington, New Zealand.

Bardach E (1998). *Getting Agencies to Work Together: The Practice and Theory of Managerial Craftmanship*. Washington, DC: Brookings Institution Press.

Barry M, Jenkins R (2007). *Implementing Mental Health Promotion*. Churchill Livingstone Elsevier.

Brewis R K, Hurford H (2004). *A Framework for Primary Mental Health Care*. East Leeds Primary Care Trust: Clements Henderson.

Brownie S (2007). *From Policy to Practice: The New Zealand Experience in Implementing Partnership-based Local Development Policy*. NSW, Australia: Faculty of Business, Charles Sturt University.

Burke D, Herrman H, Evans M, Cockram A (2000). Educational aims for trainees and supervisors in multidisciplinary teams. *Australasian Psychiatry* **8**, 336–339.

Chrislip D (2002). *The Collaborative Leadership Fieldbook: A Guide for Citizens and Civic Leaders*. San Francisco: Jossey-Bass.

Coffee R, Jones G (2000). Why should anyone be led by you? *Harvard Business Review* Sept-Oct, 63–70.

Considine M (1994). *Public Policy: A Critical Approach*. Melbourne: Macmillan Education Australia Pty Ltd.

Considine M (2004). *Changing the Way Government Works*. Melbourne: IPAA Victoria.

Craven M, Bland R (2006). Better practices in collaborative mental health care: an analysis of the evidence base. *Canadian Journal of Psychiatry* **51**, 8–72.

D'amour D, Ferrada-Videla M, San Martin Rodriguez L, *et al.* (2005). The conceptual basis for interprofessional collaboration: core concepts and theoretical frameworks. *The Journal of Interpersonal Care* **1**, Suppl 116–131.

DuBrin A, Dalglish C (2003). *Leadership, An Australasian Focus*. Milton: John Wiley and Sons.

Emmerson B, Freidin J, Sara G, Newman L (2004). A health policy unit: why do we need one? *Australasian Psychiatry* **12**(1), 103–104.

Evans B, Joas M, Sundback S, Theobald K (2005). *Governing Sustainable Cities*. London: Earthscan.

Freidin J A (2002). *Policy Development Proposal*. Melbourne: The Royal Australian and New Zealand College of Psychiatrists.

Friedli L, Parsonage M (2007). *Mental Health Promotion: Building an Economic Case*. Belfast: Northern Ireland Association for Mental Health (NIAMH).

Froggatt D, Fadden G, Johnson D L, Leggatt M, Shankar R (2007). *Families as Partners in Mental Health Care: A Guidebook for Implementing Family Work*. Toronto: World Fellowship for Schizophrenia and Allied Disorders.

Frydman B, Wilson I, Wyer J (2000). *The Power of Collaborative Leadership: Lessons for the Learning Organization*. Boston: Butterworth-Heinemann.

Greenleaf R (1977). *Servant Leadership: A Journey into the Nature of Legitimate Power and Greatness*. New York: Paulist Press.

Grint K (ed.) (1997). *Leadership: Classical, Contemporary, and Critical Approaches*. Oxford/New York: Oxford University Press.

Hall P (2005). Interprofessional cultures as barriers. *The Journal of Interpersonal Care* **1**, Suppl 188–196.

Herrman H, Trauer T, Warnock J and the Professional Liaison Committee (Australia), RANZCP (2002). The roles and relationships of psychiatrists and other service providers in mental health services. *Australian and New Zealand Journal of Psychiatry* **36**, 75–80.

Herrman H, Saxena S, Moodie R (2005). *Promoting Mental Health: Concepts, Emerging Evidence and Practice*. Geneva: World Health Organization.

Higgs M (2002). Leadership – the Long Line: A View on How We Can Make Sense of Leadership in the 21st Century. Henley: Henley Business School, University of Reading (Henley Working Paper Series, HWP 0207).

Horby S (1993). *Collaborative Care: Interprofessional, Interagency and Interpersonal*. Oxford: Blackwell Scientific Publishing.

Hosking D (1988). Organizing, leadership, and skilful process. *Journal of Management Studies* **25**(2), 147–166.

Jackson C L, Nicholson C, *et al.* (2006). Integration, co-ordination & multidisciplinary care in Australia: growth via optimal governance arrangements. The University of Queensland, Australian Primary Health Care Research Institute.

Lomas J, Woods J, Veenstra G, *et al.* (1997). Devolving authority for health research care in Canada's provinces: an introduction to the issues. *Canadian Medical Journal* **156**, 371–377.

Macdonald E, Herrman H, Hinds P, Crowe J, McDonald P (2002). Beyond interdisciplinary boundaries: views of consumers, carers and non-government organisations on teamwork. *Australasian Psychiatry* **10**(2), 125–129.

Maj M (2009). Physical health care in persons with severe mental illness: a public health and ethical priority. *World Psychiatry* **8**(1), 1–2.

Morgan K (1997). The learning region; institutions, innovation and regional renewal. *Regional Studies* **31**, 491–503.

Newton R (2009). Values Add Value: Medical Leadership in Interesting Times. RANZCP Annual Congress, Adelaide, Australia 24 May 2009.

OECD (2006). *Successful Partnerships: A Guide*. Paris: OECD.

Patterson C (2002). *Policy Options Discussion Paper*. Melbourne: RANZCP.

Prince M, Patel V, Saxena S, *et al.* (2007). No health without mental health. *Lancet* **370**, 859–877.

RANZCP (2008). *Working with the Community: The Royal Australian and New Zealand College of Psychiatrists' Strategic Plan 2009–2011*. Melbourne: RANZCP.

Saxena S, Jané-Llopis E, Hosman C (2006). Prevention of mental and behavioural disorders: implications for policy and practice. *World Psychiatry* **5**(1), 5–14.

Schofield H, Bloch S, Herrman H, Murphy B, Nankervis J, Singh B (1998). *Family Caregivers: Disability, Illness and Ageing*. Melbourne: Allen & Unwin.

Senge P (1995). Robert Greenleaf's legacy: a new foundation for twenty-first century institutions. In L C Spears (ed.) *Reflections on Leadership*. New York: John Wiley & Sons, pp. 217–240.

Sergiovanni T (1994). Organizations or communities? Changing the metaphor changes the theory. *Education Administration Quarterly* **28**(3), 214–226.

Spears L (1995). Servant-leadership and the Greenleaf legacy. In L C Spears (ed.) *Reflections on Leadership*. New York: John Wiley and Sons, pp. 1–14.

Starr J (2001). *Leadership and Local Context: A Qualitative Case Study of Interagency Collaboration in a New Jersey Community*. New York: Graduate School of Education of Harvard University.

Stone N (2007). Coming in from the interprofessional cold in Australia. *Australian Health Review* **31**(3), 332–340.

Wheatley M (1999). *Leadership and the New Science: Discovering Order in a Chaotic World*. San Francisco: Berrett-Koehler Publishers.

WHO (2005). *WHO Resource Book on Mental Health, Human Rights and Legislation*. Geneva: World Health Organization.

Yukl G (1998). *Leadership in Organizations*. Upper Saddle River: Prentice Hall.

Professionalism and psychiatry
The way forward

Dinesh Bhugra and Amit Malik

Introduction

In the preceding chapters, we have examined various facets of the debate on professionalism in medicine and, more specifically, in psychiatry. It is now crucial that, on the basis of the discussion within this volume, we recommend some action points for the profession. Whilst there are a few significant aspects discussed below that apply specifically to psychiatry, the action plan is for the most part relevant to the whole of medicine. The core virtues of a profession are embedded in moral links, fidelity to trust, benevolence and intellectual honesty, along with courage, compassion and truthfulness (Racey 1990). Quite often these values get overlooked in a world which is increasingly consumer-oriented, and medicine starts to become a business rather than a vocation or a profession. *Phronesis* lies at the heart of professionalism. Phronesis is a Socratic concept dealing with wisdom which arguably can be gained through experience, judgement and intellectual ability and knowledge. Racey (1990) also argues that the central virtue of professionalism is practical wisdom, which unites moral and intellectual virtues. Moral values, probity and honesty remain crucial aspects of professionalism. However, the challenge is how to transmit these values to members of the profession when public trust towards a number of occupations is dwindling fairly rapidly.

Johnston's (2006) important point that professionalism is dynamic and responds to change is essential to our thinking and to the way professionalism develops in this century. Without doubt, no doctor would agree that greed, misrepresentation, abuse of power and position, breaches of confidentiality and sexual harassment (Page 2006) are acceptable in this day and age, if ever they were. Joyner and Vemulakonda (2007) emphasize that the medical profession must be guided by three principles: knowledge, trained skills and service (along with altruism) to the society in which the individuals practise. Using interventions through teaching, they reported that various components of professionalism – such as respect, compassion, commitment to ethical principles and sensitivity to diversity – can be taught. The challenge is to ensure that these values remain embedded in the individual's clinical practice. Not all components of professionalism, such as caring and compassion, can be measured, but communication skills can and should be. Stern (2004) makes some useful suggestions for measuring medical professionalism. If the core concepts of professionalism are perceived as character, knowledge and skills, then certainly the latter two can be learnt and indeed taught (Russell 2006). With regard to the agenda for quality of care in mental health services, it is crucial that we, as professionals, lead on measuring the quality not only of the structures but also of the processes, which often get ignored in the broader scheme of things.

Professionalism in Mental Healthcare: Experts, Expertise and Expectations, ed. Dinesh Bhugra and Amit Malik. Published by Cambridge University Press. © Cambridge University Press 2011.

Changing with the world

In this volume, Sartorius comprehensively sets the global societal context within which professionalism is facing brand new challenges. He specifically discusses the issues of commodification of healthcare, loss of social capital and the advent of the technological revolution, which present a very new world in which medical professionalism must be exercised. The profession must take into account these global changes and undertake an urgent debate to understand their implications for healthcare delivery at a global, national and local level.

Medicine and the law: strengthening the partnership

Historically, the legal system has strongly reflected the altruistic and autonomous nature of medical professionalism, but this exalted status has recently been under greater scrutiny. There is a responsibility for medicine to be at the forefront of creating transparency within the regulatory framework and with greater involvement of patients and lay representatives in the process, not only of developing regulatory structures but also of monitoring the practice of individual doctors and the law, ensuring that medicine is free to act professionally in the service of patients and society at large.

Ethics at the heart of professionalism

As ethical principles are central to making medicine a profession, it is incumbent upon the profession to use ethics as a basis for continually renegotiating its contract with society. Modern medical ethics must place patient welfare at the heart of any debate regarding the changing relationship between the profession and society at large.

Professionalism and expertise

Attaining and maintaining medical expertise are core to the trust bestowed upon physicians by society and are key not only to the doctor–patient relationship but to professionalism in general. The medical profession must put structures in place that allow novice undergraduate medical students to develop into experts, as well as ensuring that experts continually maintain their professional expertise. Additionally, it is the responsibility of each medical professional to acquire and then maintain this expertise and use this as the basis for the care of their patients. The distinction between the expert and the professional is important (see Bhugra and Gupta 2010a for further discussion).

Putting patients before self

Reviewing the history of medical professionalism in most developed countries, it is very clear that the medical profession is strongest when it leads the movement for patient welfare, even if it is at the expense of professional autonomy. Therefore, from time to time the medical profession must engage in introspection and self-examination, unprompted by external influences, in order to ensure that it is prioritizing patient and societal welfare over self-interest.

New professionalism: relationships, teamworking and leadership

The concept of new professionalism is very much focused on relationships and collaboration. The most central amongst all possible relationships within this context is the relationship between the healthcare professional and the patient. The profession must use this relationship as the foundation for wider relationships, such as the physician–other healthcare professionals, the physician–society and the physician–self relationships. Psychiatric professionals in particular must be able to develop a relationship with the patient that is based on caring, trust and respect for patient autonomy and welfare.

New professionalism must view effective teamworking as crucial to its existence and development, especially in psychiatry, where high-quality and holistic patient care can only be delivered by a well-functioning multidisciplinary team. The role of teams can and should extend to supporting the health and welfare of other clinical team members, as maintaining one's own health is crucial for any physician in order for them to serve their patients.

The concept of professionalism and collaboration must also extend to the psychiatrist's relationship with and leadership within the wider society. 'New professionalism' must incorporate a collaborative model where psychiatrists work in teams and provide distributed leadership within the context of interagency and interprofessional collaboration. A part of their professional role must also extend to working in collaboration with and providing leadership to the local communities, in such sectors as primary healthcare, education, the criminal justice system and employment, as an expert on mental health issues in these sectors.

Collaborations, relationships and leadership roles must be contextualized within the socio-economic and cultural milieu in which a psychiatrist practises. For instance, the role of specialists in resource-poor settings, in addition to providing one-to-one patient care, must also be one of collaboration and leadership in supporting mental health programmes, carrying out priority research, building capacity and leading in mental health advocacy (see Bhugra and Gupta 2010b).

In addition to the roles of individual professionals, professional associations are well placed to work with policy-makers in the development of mental health policies that affect populations as a whole. National and international psychiatric organizations and societies must contribute to public mental health policy and establish partnerships with external stakeholders, such as national governments and international health organizations like the World Health Organization. Organizations and societies that do not shift their focus outwards but continue to focus solely on their members' interests are likely to become increasingly less relevant in a world of 'new' professionalism, where there is primacy of patient welfare over physician interests. Bhugra (2009) has found that a large proportion of trainees and trained psychiatrists believe the values of professionalism should be dealt with by the profession itself and by professional organizations.

Teaching professionalism

Medicine and psychiatry must continue to build on the initial work undertaken, at least in the Anglo-Saxon world, towards the formal teaching of professionalism and its assessment. Whilst much emphasis is placed on the teaching of medical professionalism in the undergraduate years, developing and maintaining medical professionalism require lifelong learning, and equal emphasis must be placed on this continuing professional development. Various aspects of professionalism, including communication, ethics and patient-centred medicine, must be taught to all medical students. The importance of assessing professional behaviours and professionalism cannot be over-emphasized, as it drives learning to be a 'professional'. It is very important to identify unprofessional behaviour early in a medical career, as there is sufficient evidence from the regulatory bodies that this is a predictor of poor professionalism in future practice and of future disciplinary proceedings. Additionally, developing and maintaining professionalism should be seen as an activity that extends throughout the professional life of a physician, and adequate arrangements should be made for this.

One of the biggest challenges facing the teaching of professionalism is the hidden curriculum, where students learn from role models, as this often promotes the learning of unprofessional attitudes and behaviours. Moreover, very few programmes actually teach attitudes towards professionalism, and there is very little evidence of interventions that induce changes in such attitudes. Finally, the formal teaching of aspects of professionalism can be seen by some as pious platitudes or powerless ideals (see Chapter 13). This stresses the importance of the honest reflection of real-life clinical and professional dilemmas as a method for promoting ethical professionalism. Psychiatry and medicine must overcome these challenges to ensure the development of undergraduate medical students into young medical professionals.

Like most things, components of professionalism can be learnt and retained using a number of different models. Of these, mentoring and apprenticeship are one approach. There are of course disadvantages to this approach in that if the mentor is not right, then a lot of wrong things can be learnt. Cruess (2006) emphasizes that to teach professionalism, various additional factors are necessary – e.g. institutional support, environment processes such as experiential learning, and role modelling by seniors and other members of the team. Furthermore, it is inevitable that individual traits such as cognitive base and personality will also play a role in this process. Cruess suggests that narrative medicine, spirituality and communication can be used in teaching professionalism.

However, learning about professionalism should start much earlier. The selection of students at both undergraduate and postgraduate levels is crucial in developing medical professionalism in the twenty-first century. It is possible that not all attitudes can be changed or learnt, but some can and should be encouraged to change. The key challenge to the profession is how to maximize the positive aspects of professionalism in the twenty-first century.

Talbott and Mallott (2006) suggest that psychiatrists are best placed to teach other medical professions about professionalism, as they have the skills and the understanding of cultures, organizations and group dynamics. They can co-ordinate components of comprehensive healthcare delivery. In addition, they have the ability to understand and adhere to ethical practice, and are able to communicate and work with patients and their families (and deal with uncertainty and ambiguity). Interviewing techniques and group work, models of public health and bioethics and hospice care professionalism and humanism can be explained and taught. Knapp (2006) recommends that patient surveys and employer valuations can provide a clue to the levels of professionalism. However, in psychiatry, patient surveys, especially among patients detained against their will or patients with dementia, may not provide an entirely accurate picture.

Facing challenges head on

There are many challenges and threats to contemporary professionalism in psychiatry. These include individual threats, such as some psychiatrists promoting self-interest over patient welfare, instances of conflicts of interest with psychiatrists and the pharmaceutical industry, the struggle to develop and maintain expertise and professionalism and the rare but very public scandals resulting from a psychiatrist's lack of probity. However, there are bigger systemic threats that confront psychiatry as we enter a new decade. These include the debates on self-versus external regulation, mandatory requirements for all psychiatrists to periodically prove their expertise, the changing role of psychiatrists within multiprofessional teams and the delivery of high-quality patient care in difficult economic times. Psychiatry will only emerge stronger as a profession if it leads the charge on all these debates with one primary principle – the welfare of our patients.

Conclusions

There are many different fronts on which the debate on professionalism within psychiatry will continue to take place. However, there are a few clear priority actions that the global psychiatric community must urgently take to promote professionalism within psychiatry. First, there must be a clear commitment from all institutions involved in undergraduate medical education, postgraduate psychiatric training and continuing professional development for career psychiatrists to support the teaching and maintenance of professionalism throughout a psychiatrist's professional career. Second, the profession should lead the charge for greater patient and lay involvement in teaching, training, service delivery and regulation within mental health services in general and in psychiatry in particular. Third, professional societies and associations, rather than focusing on the needs of their members, must engage with policy-makers at a national and international level to improve and enhance the delivery of care to all those suffering from mental illnesses. Finally, the profession as a whole needs to work with the legal systems and employers to ensure a new form of professional autonomy – one that allows psychiatrists to deliver the high-quality care that society expects of them.

References

Bhugra D (2009). Professionalism and psychiatry: the profession speaks. *Acta Psychiatrica Scandinavica* **118**, 327–329.

Bhugra D, Gupta S (2010a). Teaching and learning professional values. *Asia Pacific Psychiatry* **2**, 65–67.

Bhugra D, Gupta S (2010b). Leadership, decision making and errors: cultural factors. *International Psychiatry* **7**(2), 27–29.

Cruess R L (2006). Teaching professionalism. *Clinical Orthopaedics and Related Research* **449**, 177–185.

Johnston G (2006). See one, do one, teach one: developing professionalism across the generations. *Clinical Orthopaedics and Related Research* **449**, 186–192.

Joyner B D, Vemulakonda V M (2007). Improving professionalism: making the implicit more explicit. *Journal of Urology* **177**, 2289–2293.

Knapp R (2006). The challenges of teaching professionalism. *Annals of Emergency Medicine* **48**, 538–539.

Page D W (2006). Professionalism and team care in the clinical setting. *Clinical Anatomy* **19**, 468–472.

Racey J (1990). Professionalism: sane and insane. *Journal of Clinical Psychology* **51**, 138–140.

Russell T R (2006). From my perspective. *Bulletin of the American College of Surgeons* **91**, 4.

Stern D T (2004). *Measuring Medical Professionalism*. New York: Oxford University Press.

Talbott J A, Mallott D B (2006). Professionalism, medical humanism and clinical bioethics: the new wave – does psychiatry have a role? *Journal of Psychiatric Practice* **12**, 384–390.

Index